BEAT DIABETES WITH INDIAN VEGETARIAN COOKING

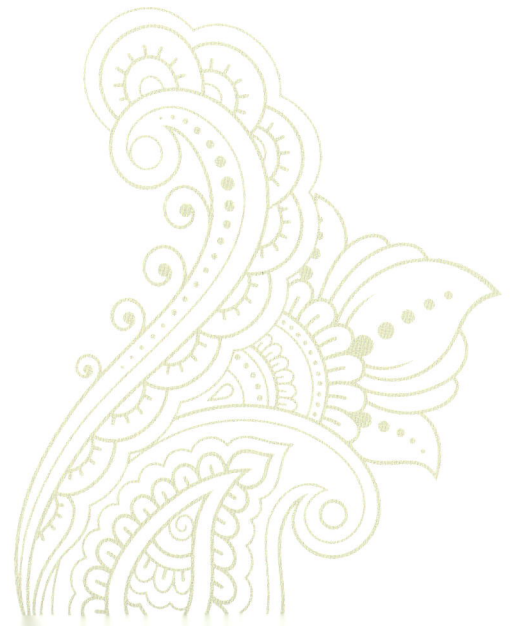

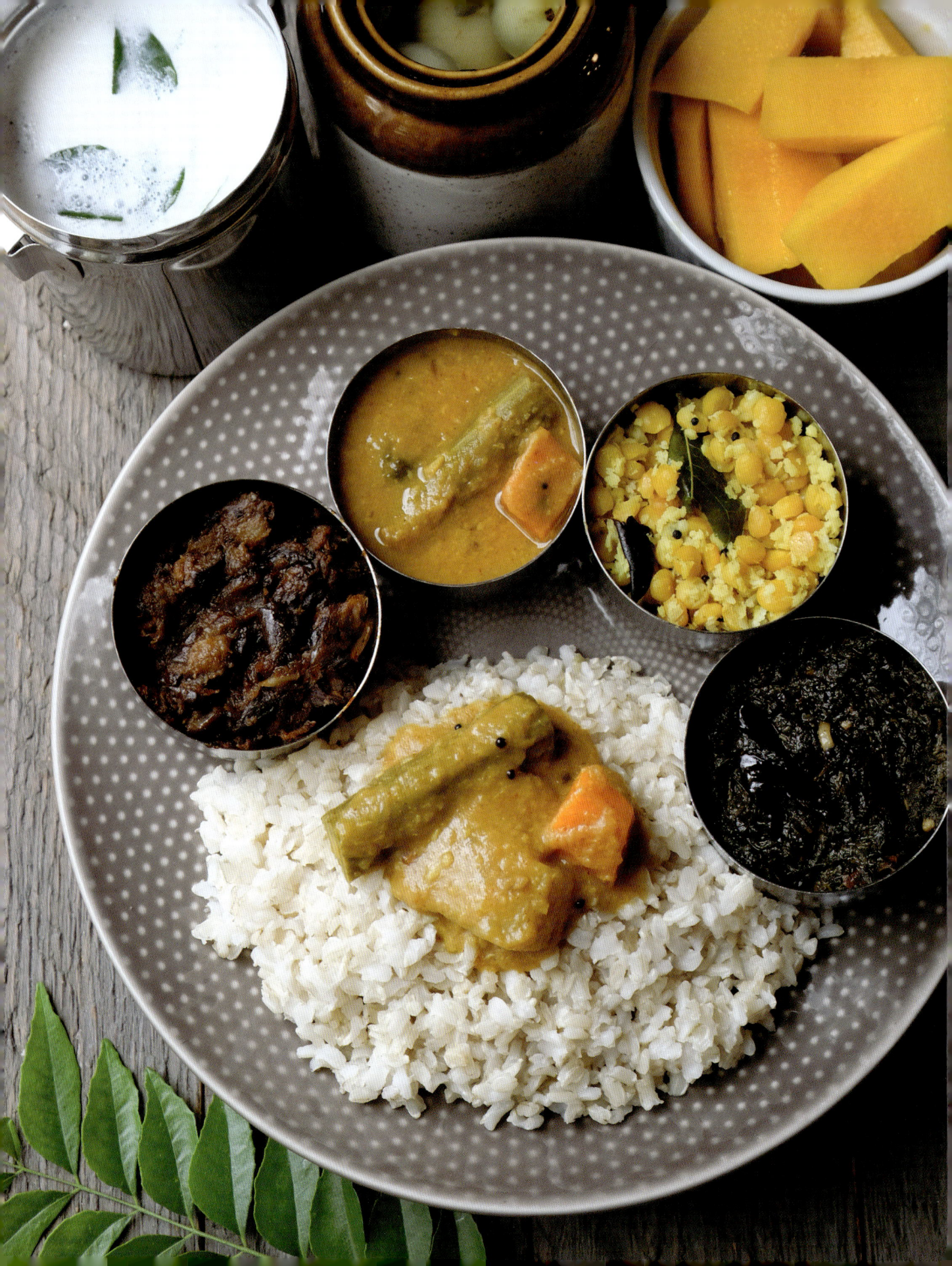

BEAT DIABETES

with

INDIAN VEGETARIAN COOKING

JOHN M. POOTHULLIL, MD, FRCP
AND D. C. HANUMANTHARAO

OVER AND ABOVE CREATIVE

Editorial Direction and Editing: Rick Benzel Creative Services

Recipes created by D. C. Hanumantharao

Creative Director: Susan Shankin/Precocity Press

Creative Consultant: Elizabeth Lenthall

Cover Design: Susan Shankin and Elizabeth Lenthall

Interior Book Design: Susan Shankin

Photography: Maya Mohan

Published by Over and Above Creative, Los Angeles, CA

ISBN: 978-0-9971077-5-3

First Edition, Printed at RRD in China

CONTENTS

PREFACE

By John Poothullil, M.D., FRCP

There may be several reasons you find yourself interested in this book. Perhaps as someone with Type 2 diabetes who is taking medications or injecting insulin, you are looking for new ways to control your blood sugar because you find it impossible to avoid the foods you love. Perhaps you have pre-diabetes and are worried about developing full-blown diabetes because some members of your family have it. Or maybe you are simply looking for a lifestyle change that will benefit your overall wellness through a vegetarian diet and exercise.

Whatever your reason for wanting to read this book, I aim to help you in two ways. First, as a retired medical doctor committed to improving people's health and overall life, I have spent more than two decades researching the medical literature to develop new insights into why people gain weight and develop high blood sugar that eventually becomes Type 2 diabetes. I will share my learnings with you in these pages, including many new ideas that can change your life. Secondly, as someone who, like most people, enjoys great tasting, healthy food, I want to offer all those who love to cook (as well as those who just love to eat what someone else cooks) recipes to make and enjoy delicious dishes that will keep your blood sugar low so you can avoid or even reverse Type 2 diabetes.

Since 2015, I have published four books detailing my insights into the real cause and the right cure for Type 2 diabetes: the modern diet full of carbohydrates, *particularly grains and grain-flour products*. My books explain the science-based theory I developed that a high-carb diet causes a normal body metabolism—muscle cells burning fatty acids rather than glucose—to go haywire. When this "fatty acid burn switch" occurs on a regular basis over years, it leaves glucose in the bloodstream, leading to high blood sugar and eventually Type 2 diabetes. I will explain more about this science shortly.

Over the years, many people asked me to write a cookbook that would help them prepare meals that keep their blood sugar low. In 2023, I teamed up with professional chef Colleen Cackowski to publish *The Diabetes-Free Cookbook and Exercise Guide*, which offered more than 80 mostly grain-free recipes for breakfasts, lunches, dinners, snacks, and desserts. In that book, we included recipes that contained various meats such as chicken, fish, and beef, along with dishes that did not include meat.

What happened next did not surprise me. Many people asked if I could publish another cookbook, this one based on fully vegetarian recipes that keep one's blood sugar low. I know there are many ways to prepare vegetarian meals. However, having grown up in Kerala, India, I immediately realized that the best vegetarian cuisine comes from my home country. The reason I say this, as you will learn from the meals suggested in this book, is that the traditional vegetarian meals in India are loaded with macronutrients, micronutrients, minerals, antioxidants, fiber, and trace elements. These are all requirements of a diverse diet that keeps you healthy because they supply your cells with a wide range of nutrients and build your immune system.

The great American chef and food lover, Anthony Bourdain, once visited India for a taping of his renowned TV show and remarked that India was one of the only places in the world "where he could happily eat vegetarian food without noticing it." He praised Indian food for its colors, textures, and spices.

Not being a chef myself, I was lucky to be acquainted with Mr. D. C. Hanumantharao of Andhra Pradesh, India who happened to be a new resident of Oregon where I live. Mr. Rao (as he likes to be called) is a retired professor of English and college principal, who had translated my book, *Diabetes—The Real Cause and the Right Cure: Eight Steps to Reverse Diabetes in Eight Weeks* into Telugu and arranged for it to be published in India. He had also translated several of my articles on diabetes and participated with me in many TV interviews on diabetes for audiences in India.

When I learned that he is not only a Sanskrit scholar but also an expert in preparing Indian vegetarian dishes based on ancient recipes written in Sanskrit centuries ago, when Type 2 diabetes was almost non-existent, I reached out and asked if he would assist me in writing this book. He excitedly agreed and proceeded to put his heart and soul into crafting 112 mouth-watering, flavorful vegetarian meals that are delicious, nutritious, and fun to make.

There are four unique elements that set this cookbook apart from many others. First is that we have created a wide variety of truly vegetarian meals, snacks, and desserts based on traditional Indian recipes, some of which literally go back thousands of years. These dishes are more than just super tasty; they are also attractive to your eyes with their colorful ingredients and to your nose with their mesmerizing aromas due to their many spices. Once you try these recipes, you will see that you can indeed eat great meals while at the same time keeping your blood sugar in check. The key is to eat foods that do not cause your blood sugar to spike so high that it takes hours to return to the normal blood sugar range. That is how you begin moving away from being prediabetic or fully diabetic. With recipes like these, you can even begin to lower your blood sugar enough to reverse a case of diagnosed Type 2 diabetes.

A second unique element is that Mr. Rao solved the key problem with traditional Indian vegetarian lunch planning: the time it takes to prepare many dishes made with many ingredients. He found a clever way to get around this by crafting what he calls a Superfast Lunch (or dinner) that can be prepared in under one hour and can be varied in different ways, as you will see in the book.

The third distinguishing element of this book is that I have included 12 simple and brief exercises that you can do to keep your body in condition. Changing your diet is the major key to avoiding Type 2 diabetes, but exercise is also important to keep your body in shape and stay flexible as you age. I know of no other cookbook that takes this holistic approach to health, considering both diet and exercise.

The fourth element that sets this book apart is that we have published it for an international audience. The reason for this is that the entire world must become far more concerned about what is becoming a global pandemic of Type 2 diabetes. The incidence of Type 2 diabetes has been rising in nearly every developed nation and even in undeveloped nations. The World Health Organization estimated that over 800 million people have diabetes, 90% of whom are Type 2 diabetics. China, India, and the U.S. in that order lead the world in the sheer number of citizens diagnosed with Type 2 diabetes. But many other nations have high rates of Type 2 diabetes as well, including Pakistan, Kuwait, Egypt, Japan, Bangladesh, Mexico, Brazil, Indonesia, Columbia, Chile, Argentina, Venezuela, as well as Guatemala, Uruguay, Puerto Rico, and Honduras.

The point is, even though these recipes are based on Indian cuisine, they are for everyone, no matter where you live, as long as you can read English. Even if you have never cooked Indian dishes before, with their unique Indian cooking methods, ingredients, and spices, you can easily learn how to make every recipe in this book no matter what your cooking skills are or what country you live in. In today's global world, you can find the Indian ingredients and spices for these recipes in many major supermarkets or in specialty Indian and Asian grocery stores.

How I Became Interested in Diabetes and What I Found Out

I am a retired medical doctor, having practiced for 35 years. I did not practice endocrinology, the medical specialty that deals with diabetes. But that allowed me to study diabetes from a different perspective and champion a different methodology for people to avoid or reverse it.

While I was in medical school, endocrinology professors told us to believe, as they did themselves, that Type 2 diabetes is a hormonal disease caused by "insulin resistance." I had no reason to dispute this.

Towards the end of my training, I became aware of one of my relatives who was diagnosed with Type 2 diabetes. She was taking insulin to control her blood sugar. Her husband, a professor in a medical school, adjusted her insulin dosage to keep her blood sugar level within an acceptable range. Nevertheless, a few years later, she had to have one of her legs amputated due to reduced blood supply to her leg—a well-known complication of Type 2 diabetes in many adults. I thought her doctor would change her diabetes medication because taking insulin had not stopped her leg complication. To my surprise though, her doctor continued the same line of treatment using insulin. Within a few more months, she had to have the other leg amputated.

I started paying more attention to people who were on insulin to treat their Type 2 diabetes. To my shock, I found others who suffered severe consequences. One friend who was a trained scientist had to have three toes amputated, one after another, after keeping his blood sugar level within normal limits for years using insulin. I soon learned about similar experiences among many acquaintances who lost their vision and others who lost kidney function.

I wondered how this could be. Despite taking medications or injecting insulin, I saw that diabetic patients still suffered the consequences of long-term diabetes. About 25 years ago, I began intently studying the medical literature on hunger, weight gain, obesity, and diabetes.

Through my research, I came to a surprising conclusion—the theory of *"insulin resistance"* was illogical and remained scientifically unproven. I knew I was going against tradition. This theory, however, is what endocrinologists believe in and is the rationale they use to keep prescribing medications and insulin injections to diabetic patients.

So, I wondered what might actually cause high blood sugar and diabetes?

I soon came to realize that the answer is staring us right in the face. It is, as I mentioned above, our modern diet, heavily filled with complex carbohydrates that flood the bloodstream with glucose (sugar). Among the many cuisines and cultures around the world, the modern diet is the only common denominator that can possibly explain the global increase in the incidence of high blood sugar and Type 2 diabetes. I do not believe that more and more humans are evolving to be insulin resistant. The body produces over 50 hormones, so why would it become resistant to just one? I also know that no genetic defect has ever been discovered that links to Type 2 diabetes.

I suggest that we can trace the rising incidence of diabetes to the "Green Revolution" of the 1960s. At this time, new technologies and fertilizers increased the farming of cultivated grains, and governments around the world began subsidizing grain production to ensure enough food for their populations. New milling technologies and lower shipping costs made grain-flour products cheap and easily available. Americans especially, but also people in most Western nations, as well as Indians began consuming a variety of breads, cakes, pooris, pasta, rice, corn, pizza, Mysore bondas, sabudana dishes, and many other foods made with rice, wheat and corn—and the list goes on.

Why Do Grains and Grain-flour Products Cause Diabetes?

Let me explain why I suggest that our modern diet high in grains and grain-flour products is the most likely trigger for the development of pre-diabetes or Type 2 diabetes. It is because the typical diet that includes more than 50% of one's daily caloric intake in the form of complex carbohydrates produces a voluminous amount of glucose that the body's cells cannot use on an immediate basis. Some glucose is stored in the liver, then released between meals for the body's energy needs until the next meal.

But here is the key—any unused glucose is transformed into fatty acids that are then stored in one's fat cells. The problem is, every individual has only a certain capacity for fat storage, based on their body type and genetic inheritance. At some point, one's fat cells can literally become full, leaving nowhere for the fatty acids produced from the unused glucose after each meal to be stored.

The result is that the fatty acids remain circulating in the bloodstream. What diabetes specialists seldom admit, however, is that our muscle cells—the largest energy producers in the body—are like a hybrid car. They can burn either glucose or fatty acids for producing energy. Fatty acids can enter right into muscle cells faster and more easily than glucose—and they do, leaving glucose in the bloodstream, thus high blood sugar.

This is what I call the *fatty acid burn switch*. A long-term diet high in complex carbohydrates is what eventually causes chronic high blood sugar—and that eventually becomes Type 2 diabetes.

As you might imagine, a diet high in grains and grain-flour products that produce excessive amounts of fatty acids that fill your fat cells is also what leads to weight gain and, for an increasing number of people, obesity. This explains why the majority of people with Type 2 diabetes are overweight or obese as they enter their 40s, 50s, and 60s. But this same diet also explains why we now see millions of children as young as 12 and teens become overweight, obese, and even diabetic.

Diabetes can also occur in thin people, simply because they have a small number of fat cells, which leaves them no room to store excess fatty acids. They too can undergo the fatty acid burn switch, creating high blood sugar and diabetes. In many developing countries, such as India, an increasing number of people are not considered to be extremely overweight, yet they develop high blood sugar and Type 2 diabetes. In some Western countries, 15% of people with Type 2 diabetes are not considered overweight.

The same biological mechanism of the fatty acid burn switch also explains why a pregnant woman with no previous history of diabetes can develop gestational diabetes. Simply put, when a pregnant woman fills up her fat storage capacity, her muscles switch to burning fatty acids, leaving glucose in the bloodstream. This explanation is in contrast to the present situation, in which endocrinologists have absolutely no hypothesis to explain the development of "insulin resistance" in lean or pregnant diabetics.

Support for Why Diet–Not Medication–Is the Key to Moderating Diabetes

Here is something odd that supports what I am telling you about the real cause of high blood sugar and diabetes. You will often hear that today's physicians recommend that people with diabetes eat a low carbohydrate diet. This advice comes from mainstream endocrinologists who still believe in the insulin resistance theory. This strikes me as odd. On one hand they recognize that a low-carb diet plays an important role in controlling high blood sugar, though they don't know why. Meanwhile, on the other hand, they tell their patients to continue taking diabetes medications or injecting insulin.

In my view, these doctors are still counting on medications as the answer to controlling blood sugar; and they are doing so only because the insulin resistance theory is what they learned in medical school. They are unable to admit this theory is wrong, yet they accept a clear connection between a low carbohydrate diet and low blood sugar.

I am not suggesting that you cannot achieve a low blood sugar level using medications. You can, at least for a while. But what I am saying is that the medication/insulin injection approach has two serious flaws.

First, it is difficult to maintain a certain desired blood glucose level using medications such as insulin. Your blood sugar level is actually a moving target. Throughout the day, and especially after each meal, it changes depending on what you eat. It swings upwards for about two hours after you eat a meal, and then slowly descends. This forces someone with high blood sugar to keep measuring the level of their blood glucose. This is why diabetics who inject insulin must decide how much insulin to inject before and after each meal, or even throughout the day.

The second flaw is what I told you about above concerning the people I knew who lost limbs or eyesight due to diabetes. There is absolutely no doubt any longer that, despite taking diabetes medications or injecting insulin, a very large percentage of diabetics still end up with one or more of the serious consequences of diabetes: loss of kidney function (which leads to permanent dialysis), loss of vision, and/or nerve damage to limbs (which results in amputation of toes or legs). Yet endocrinologists still prefer to treat diabetes using medications or insulin injections rather than emphasizing to their patients that *they must alter their diet*. This is tragic.

For these reasons, I suggest that it is far better to control your blood sugar level by regulating what you eat. Let me put it this way: if you don't put glucose (carbohydrates) into your mouth, you won't need to worry about having high blood sugar. Doesn't this make logical sense to you? The fact is that cultivated grains or foods made with them are not necessary for healthy living.

You may not completely understand the science behind what I have just explained. But that is okay. If you want to learn more about that science, click on the QR code to see an animation video titled "Challenging Your Assumptions about Type 2 Diabetes" that illustrates the concept of the fatty acid burn switch. You can also read more about "authentic weight," weight gain, and obesity in my book, *Beat Unwanted Weight Gain: 7 Ways to Lose Pounds and Never Regain Them.*

.

Try These Recipes for Just One Month

For now, what counts most is recognizing that *your diet is the single most important factor you can control to lower your blood sugar*—and even potentially to prevent or reverse Type 2 diabetes. If you are willing to try altering your diet using some of these recipes for just a few weeks, you will see your blood sugar level go down, you may lose a few pounds, and you will feel healthier and more active.

The greatest advantage of these recipes is that you will not lose your enjoyment of eating or be told to follow a lot of restrictions. For example, these recipes do not show how many calories are in them. My belief is that most people have enough fat stored up in their body to have the energy they need to make it through any given day. Moreover, no one can predict how many calories one may expend during a given day. Therefore, counting calories makes little sense for the average person—and most people struggle to stay within a calorie count anyway. What is more important is that we eat to acquire the nutrients the cells of the body need and that we learn to become more conscious of our eating behaviors.

Neither Mr. Rao nor I know how much of what nutrient your body needs when you sit down to eat. Your brain, on the other hand, knows what your body needs and will create the sensation of enjoyment when you consume a food that contains the needed nutrients. More importantly, your brain reduces the intensity of enjoying that food when a sufficient amount has been eaten. In my view, the more effective guideline is thus to eat whatever you enjoy but also pay attention to that level of enjoyment or loss of enjoyment. To do this, you need to chew your food thoroughly; this is necessary to release the nutrients in your mouth at a rate at which your taste buds and olfactory sensors can record and report their findings to the control centers in the brain. If you pay attention to this "enjoyment, less enjoyment" cycle, you don't need to pre-measure how much you eat.

I invite you to use this book as a steppingstone to a new lifestyle of healthy eating. Begin by using as many of the recipes as you can for just one month as a starting point. Each recipe in this cookbook is composed of ingredients that will not cause your blood sugar to elevate too high or for too long after eating. In this way, you can achieve a more stable blood sugar level throughout the day. You're bound to notice a difference in just a few weeks.

What is most important is for you to believe that you can control your blood sugar and your destiny starting right now. If you are feeling anxious about making all your meals using these recipes, do not worry. Keep the book in your kitchen as a gentle reminder and aim to use some of the recipes to make at least half your meals over the next 30 days. While perhaps not as effective as a complete overhaul of your diet would be, it will be a good start in your effort to lower your blood sugar through your diet. If you can achieve at least a modest level of blood sugar reduction in the coming 30 days, you may be encouraged to cook entirely using these recipes in the following days.

I know it is not easy for many people to give up foods they enjoy, especially those "comfort foods" they have been eating since childhood. But in general, these recipes do not ask you to give up much, other than avoiding carbohydrate-heavy meals. The main suggestion I would like to make you, wherever you live in the world, is to avoid eating the same amount of grains as you typically ate before. (Wherever you live in the world, you likely have fast-food restaurants that tempt you with high-carb foods, like thick bread sandwiches, burgers on large buns, pizza, tacos, rice dishes, cakes, Mysore bondas, and grain-flour sweets and desserts. You might want to eat far fewer of these foods!) I assure you: you won't starve making these recipes, because we have included meals and desserts that will give you the same feeling of satisfaction as you are used to. Perhaps even more.

You may make some mistakes or experience anxiety about changing your food preferences. You may find yourself slipping and backsliding multiple times, returning to consuming fast foods and grain-based snacks, especially when you are sharing a meal with family and friends who prompt you to eat what they enjoy. You may cave in and give up on trying these recipes, accepting that your life will be easier if you just keep taking your medication to control your blood sugar. You may find it hard to ignore that your past attempts of dietary changes did not help you to accomplish your goal.

Your feeling this way is understandable because a fundamental change in your dietary practices is often painful and challenging to sustain. You may have come to believe that because of your family history—other family members who have diabetes—that you are not likely to escape diabetes for the rest of your life.

However, keep in mind that science has not found any genetic cause for Type 2 diabetes. Meanwhile, my hypothesis is supported by scientific, logical evidence, that the modern carbohydrate-heavy diet is what triggers high blood sugar and diabetes.

At moments when you are feeling hesitant and apprehensive about making the dietary changes I suggest, remember that the best guarantee of preserving the functions of your kidneys, preventing heart attacks, maintaining your brain function, keeping your eyesight, and avoiding amputation of your limbs is by controlling your blood sugar through lifestyle changes—particularly your diet—rather than by resorting to a lifetime of medications such as insulin. I assure you that as you take control of what you can accomplish on your own, many of the fears of a recurrence of demoralizing dietary failures of the past will vanish and you will feel emboldened.

Add These 12 Simple Exercises to Create a New Lifestyle

As I said earlier, a complementary component of this cookbook is a set of twelve simple exercises you can do in the comfort of your own home or anywhere. I chose to include these because people with Type 2 diabetes are often adults who do not exercise enough relative to their age. Let's face it: as we age, we're no longer "spring chickens," full of enough energy to exercise an hour or more each day. In fact, the older we get, the harder it is to burn calories as we did when we were younger. Most older adults lose muscle mass (notice, for instance, how your leg muscles are thinner). This means that a half hour of exercise for a man or woman older than 40 burns far fewer calories than for a man or woman younger than 40.

To go along with the printed exercise instructions in this book, I also produced a series of animated videos that show you how to do these twelve movements. While you may prefer to do physical activity outdoors—such as walking, running, cycling, or swimming—those can be challenging for a lot of people, especially if you are busy, or the weather conditions don't allow it, or if you are confined to your home for any reason. I thus developed this set of twelve easy-to-do exercises that you can do inside your own home at any time.

For example, if you find you are bored or when you are just sitting around on the couch, you can do the deep breathing exercise, paying attention to the movement of air through your nose and the movement of your chest wall muscles. It's a great exercise to do when you are watching TV as well, especially to pass the time during commercials.

Toe taps are an excellent activity when you are a passenger in a car, train, or airplane, or when there is a dull moment while you are sitting and watching a stage or sporting event, during a meeting, or while waiting for an appointment. You could also do toe taps in the standing position when you are forced to stand in a train or subway car, or any slow-moving commuter vehicle, using one leg after another.

You can do the leg-related exercises every morning before you get out of your bed. In fact, every time you lie down, you have an opportunity to do one or more of the leg exercises.

If you have a history of feeling dizzy when you stand up suddenly after being on your back for some time, this could be due to a condition called postural hypotension. Doing leg exercises before getting up to a sitting position or doing toe tapping in the sitting position before standing up, could speed delivery of blood to your brain and limit the degree of dizziness from postural hypotension.

Over time, you may find other opportunities to put these exercises into practice.

Organization of the Book

Part 1 of this book includes a brief introduction from Mr. D.C. Hanumantharao, followed by the recipes. Each recipe includes the list of ingredients to use when cooking, followed by the specific cooking directions.

Part 2 provides written explanations for how to do the exercises. Each exercise has a QR code that you can capture with your phone's camera; it will take you right to a page on the internet where you can watch the animated video showing you how to perform that exercise.

PART 1

112 TEMPTING RECIPES TO SUPPORT BLOOD SUGAR CONTROL

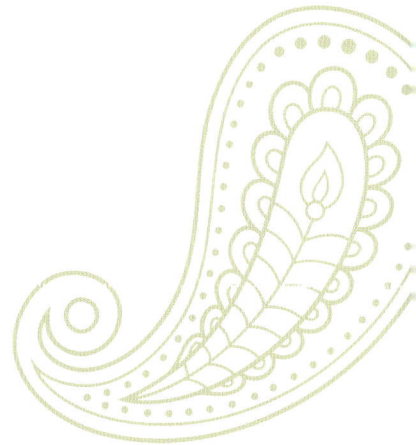

INTRODUCTION
by D.C. Hanumantharao

"The treatment of human diseases should be done in the kitchen, but not in hospital."

—CHARAKA, the Father of the Ayurvedic
system of Indian medicine, 300 B.C.

This insight suggests that the first step to addressing a health issue should focus on dietary changes and healthy eating habits at home, rather than seeking medical intervention, resulting in the use of medicines and their concomitant side effects. The approach using drugs often causes not only damage to the vital systems and organs of the body but the loss of money.

This same idea has been advocated by Dr. John Poothullill, M.D., who in his book, *Diabetes: The Real Cause and the Right Cure,* emphasizes the power of a good diet in preventing and controlling Type 2 diabetes through a shift from grain-based foods to non-grain foods. Dr. John's rationale and strong conviction motivated me to create what you will find in this book—112 incredibly delicious diabetes-friendly meals.

While translating Dr. John's book on diabetes last year, I became totally convinced by his contention that Type 2 diabetes is a lifestyle condition, not an endocrinology disease. This means you can reverse this type of diabetes through foods that do not cause spikes in your blood sugar levels, supplemented with physical activity like walking and other exercise. Dr. John sincerely pleads for a diet mostly free from grains like rice, wheat, and corn, all of which are full of complex carbohydrates that create high blood sugar levels. Over time, a diet high in carbohydrates causing high blood sugar will lead to Type 2 diabetes. Instead, Dr. John advocates a largely non-grain diet, which will not only control high blood sugar, but prevent the onset of Type 2 diabetes, a chronic disease that deteriorates your quality of life.

Given this background, I embarked on the task of crafting a large number of vegetarian dishes that are capable of not only controlling diabetes, but also providing exceptional taste experiences and real enjoyment. I have created 112 recipes, including breakfasts, lunches, dinners, snacks, sweets, salads, and dressings based on traditional Indian cuisine, some elements of which date back hundreds of years in cookbooks written in Sanskrit.

All the dishes for which I have created recipes are traditional Indian vegetarian dishes, but prepared with various millets, quinoa, oats, cauliflower rice, and brown rice in place of the usual grains like wheat and white rice, which trigger higher blood sugar levels. Many types of vegetables, beans, lentils, and leafy vegetables are also main ingredients in many recipes. In addition, my recipes utilize a large number of spices, herbs, and seeds, which not only add to the taste of the dishes, but further promote their healthful properties and diabetes-friendly nature.

The Glycemic Index

Before you start reading the recipes, here is some information about why the ingredients in these recipes do not raise your blood sugar as high as other common ingredients used in many national cuisines. You may not have heard about what is called the "glycemic index." This is a ranking of foods based on how fast they raise blood sugar. Foods are categorized as either low, medium or high. Here are some examples:

- **Low 1 to 55:** green vegetables, many fruits, raw carrots, kidney beans, chickpeas, and lentils.

- **Medium 56 to 69:** honey, bananas, pineapple, raisins, cherries, multigrain, and whole-grain wheat.

- **High 70 to 100:** white rice, white bread, potatoes, and rice-, wheat-, and corn-flour based foods.

The recipes in this book largely use low-glycemic index ingredients, which is why they are diabetes-friendly.

Getting to Know the Ingredients

If you have never cooked Indian cuisine before or you are a novice at cooking even though you live in India, here is a list of ingredients I use in the dishes in this book that you might want to become familiar with. I have shaped the recipes in this book around these ingredients because they help maintain healthy blood sugar levels. The explanations below will clarify many questions people often have about these ingredients and why they are used in Indian cuisine.

- **Ajwain:** Contains fiber, antioxidants, and other beneficial nutrients. Health benefits include controlling blood sugar levels, cholesterol, and indigestion.

- **Asafetida:** A savory enhancer that helps in managing blood sugar levels in the human body. Aids digestion and helps control bronchitis.

- **Beetroot:** Promotes cardiovascular health. Its antioxidant nature prevents cell damage and inflammation, offering protection against cancer and heart disease. It also contains healthy fats, minerals and vitamins.

- **Beans:** Contain protein, fiber, minerals, and antioxidants. Protect gut health, control blood pressure, and help in blood sugar regulation.

- **Black pepper:** Has antioxidant and anti-inflammatory properties, potentially reducing chronic disease risk. A good source of manganese, a mineral that can help with bone health, wound healing, and metabolism.

- **Cardamom:** Has many health benefits like digestive health, blood sugar and blood pressure control, and weight management. Also has antioxidant and anti-inflammatory properties.

- **Cauliflower:** High in vitamins C and K and also contains many minerals. A good source of fiber which can help with digestion and weight management. Also contains low amount of carbohydrate and so it effectively controls blood sugar.

- **Chili:** Contains many beneficial compounds, including capsaicin, vitamin C, and potassium, which helps with cancer prevention, heart health, digestion, immune system, and blood pressure.

- **Chickpeas:** High in selenium, magnesium, potassium, vitamin B, fiber, and iron. Support heart health and prevent high blood pressure.

- **Coconut:** Contains fiber, antioxidants, minerals, healthy fats and nutrients. Supports blood sugar control, and prevents infections related to root canals and other teeth issues.

- **Cumin seed:** Rich in antioxidants, which help prevent diseases like cancer, heart disease, and high blood pressure. Helps with digestion and improves blood sugar control. Also aids weight loss. Also has many antimicrobial properties.

- **Coriander seed:** Has many health benefits, including helping digestion, blood sugar and blood pressure control, and promoting heart health. Rich in antioxidants to help prevent various diseases.

- **Carrots:** Fiber in carrots can help control blood sugar levels. Loaded with vitamin A and beta carotene. Can lower diabetes risk.

- **Dates:** Rich in nutrients, fiber, antioxidants, and have many potential health benefits, including blood sugar control and bone and brain health.

- **Fenugreek seed:** Lowers blood sugar levels and increases breast milk production. Also reduces cholesterol levels, inflammation, and has anti-diarrheal properties.

- **Ginger:** Offers many health benefits, including blood sugar control, digestive aid, improving cholesterol, strengthening the immune system, preventing cancer and giving protection against Alzheimer's disease.

- **Garlic:** Rich in antioxidants. Controls blood sugar and cholesterol. Is an anti-inflammatory and antimicrobial.

- **Leafy vegetables:** Contain fiber, which helps with digestion and blood sugar control. Rich in vitamins, minerals, antioxidants, and nutrients.

- **Lentils:** Rich in fiber, so they help in blood sugar control. Also rich in minerals, proteins, and fiber to promote all-round health.

- **Mustard seed:** A good source of several vitamins, including C and K, thiamine, riboflavin, vitamin B6 and folic acid. Rich in antioxidants.

- **Nuts:** Rich in fiber, proteins, and minerals. Promote overall health, blood sugar control, and weight loss. Have many other health benefits.

- **Oats:** A low glycemic index grain. Rich in fiber. Help control blood sugar levels. Contain many vitamins, minerals, and nutrients.

- **Onions:** Rich in antioxidants and anti-cancer and anti-microbial compounds. Help blood sugar control, heart, bone and gut health.

- **Quinoa:** Low glycemic index pseudo-grain. Contains a good amount of vitamins, minerals, proteins, and antioxidants besides high quantity of fiber. Helps in blood sugar balance, weight management, as well as gut and heart health.

- **Radish:** Good source of fiber, vitamin C, potassium, calcium, and antioxidants. Helps control blood sugar levels and promotes overall health.

- **Tomatoes:** Rich in vitamins, antioxidants, fiber, potassium, and vitamins. Aid in controlling blood sugar levels, preventing cancer, and promoting heart health. Also promote all-round health.

- **Turmeric:** Active component, curcumin, helps lower blood sugar levels and reduce diabetes. Has anti-inflammatory, anti-cancer, antimicrobial, antiviral, and antiseptic properties.

Comparison of Grains

Here is a chart showing the various types of grains and millets with information regarding how much carbohydrate, fiber, fat and protein each one contains. This comparison will help you understand the importance of switching from your usual dishes made with white rice, corn, or wheat to those using millets, quinoa, and oats. As you can see, oats, quinoa, and millet have much lower amounts of carbohydrate, more fiber content, and more protein than white rice, wheat, and corn.

Grain	Carbohydrate	Fiber content	Fat content	Protein
White rice	91	1	1	7
Wheat	82	1.2	1.5	12.6
Corn	82	3	1	3
Oats	66	11.6	6.9	16.9
Quinoa	64	7	1.9	14.1
Millet	54	22.6	1.0	7.4

Notes on Preparing the Recipes

- All the recipes for the breakfasts, lunches, dinners, and snacks I have created are without the usual grains. In place of grains, the recipes use millets, oats, quinoa, and cauliflower rice. The only exception is the occasional use of brown rice, which has a low glycemic index and less carbohydrate content than regular rice. Still, I advise you to restrict your brown rice consumption to once a week.

- The recipes using millets, quinoa, and oats should be eaten in the same quantity as you may have eaten rice, corn, or wheat in the past. However, it is advisable that you eat the dals, curries, and vegetable stews in a larger quantity, and the lead meal— i.e., the cooked millet, quinoa, oats, etc.—in a smaller quantity.

- In India, lunch is the largest meal of the day, as it is in many countries. For this reason, I have provided a menu of recipes for the lunches that includes as many as four dishes —dal, curry, chutney and stew — plus buttermilk. You can leave out one, two, or even three of them. (As regards buttermilk, you can also leave this out if you are not in the habit of taking it, and there is no harm.) If you do not have time to make all the recipes included in a lunch menu, you can use the recipes labelled as breakfast for lunch.

- Whatever food you eat should be chewed thoroughly, as eating this way is highly beneficial in many ways to help you become more aware of when you have eaten enough.

- Among the ten dinner dishes is barley roti, though barley has a high carbohydrate content. Still, in view of its low glycemic index and high amount of fiber, I have suggested it. However, it should be limited to once a week or ten days.

- Regarding vegetables, I have included all types except potato, sweet potato, and corn, which are high in carbohydrates.

- While all fruits can happily be enjoyed, I suggest you avoid fruit juices and blended drinks made with fruits. When you drink these, they go directly into your body, where they spike your blood sugar levels. Besides, when you blend, you have no control over the amount you drink and thus tend to drink more than eating a single fruit. You also miss the chance to chew the fruit, so you tend to consume more calories. This advice to chew and eat fruits for your health is good not only for diabetics but for everyone.

- Feel free to vary the recipes as you wish. For example, I provide a different chutney to accompany each breakfast and dinner, but you can exchange them as you like. The chutney for ragi dosa can be eaten with green gram dosa, upma, or idli. Similarly, the chutneys I include with the breakfasts can be eaten with a dinner recipe as you desire, or vice versa. Likewise, sambar can be eaten, in addition to chutney, for breakfast or dinner per your taste. Similarly, any dal, curry, chutney, or stew can be eaten for any lunch.

- Some recipes utilize gluten-free foods, since many sensitive individuals cannot tolerate gluten in their digestion.

- In regard to the quantity of the vegetables such as green chilis, dry red chilis, and others that you use in preparing the dishes, I have suggested specific amounts. However, the size of many vegetables varies from place to place. So, depending on the size of the vegetables available in your area, you might want to increase or decrease the amounts I have suggested in the recipes.

- Regarding using chilis (green or red), salt, tamarind, jaggery, and lemon juice or citric acid, you can increase or decrease the quantity I suggest, depending on your taste. Similarly, I have not suggested jaggery in some recipes, but you can use it as per your taste. You can use lemons, green mangoes, star gooseberries, or green tamarind for a better advantage when it is possible for you.

- Garlic is used in some of the recipes, but it is optional. You can leave it out if you do not like it or cannot tolerate it. Similarly, jaggery is optional for some chutneys and stews as per your taste.

- For cooking oils, you can use more or less oil depending on your taste, as oil is not known to affect blood sugar levels. Recommended oils for people with diabetes in Indian cuisine are peanut oil, sesame oil, sunflower oil, and rice bran oil, and of course, ghee, which is used in some dishes instead of oil for a better taste.

- Salt should be used in moderation. In the recipes, I have suggested "a sufficient quantity" of salt, leaving it up to you to determine the amount you need for your taste. Note, however, that too much salt creates a risk of high blood pressure and can lead to dementia.

- It is best if all your family members eat the same foods I have suggested when you make a meal using the recipes in this book. This will free you from the trouble of cooking many types of food for your household while encouraging everyone to eat healthy, diabetes-friendly foods.

English and Indian Food Names

Here is a list of dals, millets, etc. with their English names and Indian equivalents for your better understanding.

English name	Indian name
Sorghum	Jowar
Finger millet	Ragi
Black gram	Urad dal
Green gram	Moong dal
Pigeon pea	Toor dal
Chickpea	Chana
Fenugreek	Methi

The Meaning of "Tempering" in the Recipes

One of the distinguishing characteristics of traditional Indian cuisine is the use of what are called "tempering ingredients." These are a combination of various ingredients that may include dry red chilis, green chilis, mustard seeds, cumin seeds, garlic, chickpea dal, black gram, asafetida, fenugreek, and curry leaves. These ingredients are roasted or fried in a small amount of oil in a small frying pan or in the same saucepan used to cook the dish. The tempering ingredients are then added to the dish to enhance its flavors before serving.

However, in some recipes, you will note that the tempering ingredients are roasted first and then the vegetables are added to them. The recipe directions will tell you exactly which tempering ingredients are used for each dish and when to roast them.

Feel free to increase or decrease the quantity of tempering ingredients I recommend, per your preference.

Note that curry leaves, green chilis, and garlic have to be roasted after the other tempering ingredients are roasted by 70%.

Cooking Equipment Needed

In India, households typically call the pot where the lead or main dish is cooked a *cooking bowl or saucepan*. In this book, we use the term saucepan. Depending on how many people you are cooking for, you might want to have several sizes of saucepans available.

Tempering ingredients are often roasted in a separate small frying pan. Alternatively, you can remove and set aside the prior ingredients that were cooked in the saucepan, then fry the tempering ingredients in the same saucepan, and finally mix them into the cooked ingredients before serving.

In many Indian recipes, ingredients are combined and ground together in a mixie, which is the equivalent of a kitchen blender or food processor. This grinding process was formerly done on a stone grinder like a mortar and pestle.

Several recipes in this book require an *idli* cooker. Idlis are small round or oval-shaped cakes that are steamed. An idli cooker is a steamer pot with one or more round trays that contain indents into which the idli batter is poured. When the pot is closed, the steam cooks the idlis.

Some recipes require a *dosa* pan, which is a large round flat pan used for making dosas, which are similar to thin pancakes, crêpes, or tortillas.

A small number of recipes require a pressure cooker.

Measurements and Serving Sizes

I have provided the measurement of ingredients for readers in any country. The recipes measure many ingredients in tablespoons and teaspoons. Some ingredients are measured in ounces (oz.), with their milliliter (ml) equivalent. Some ingredients are measured in kilos with their equivalent given in terms of pounds (lbs.).

The recipes are measured out to serve 1 person. If you are serving more people, you can multiply the ingredient quantities by the number of people.

Note: Because these recipes are intended to avoid or reverse Type 2 diabetes, many of them are based on a smaller serving size (6 ounces, 160 ml rather than 1 standard 8 ounce, 240 ml cup), especially for the lead or main meal, i.e., the millet, quinoa, etc. This is healthier for Type 2 diabetics to keep their blood sugar low. If you can, it is even better to restrict the measurement of the lead or main meal to 4 ounces, 120 ml to avoid spikes in high blood sugar.

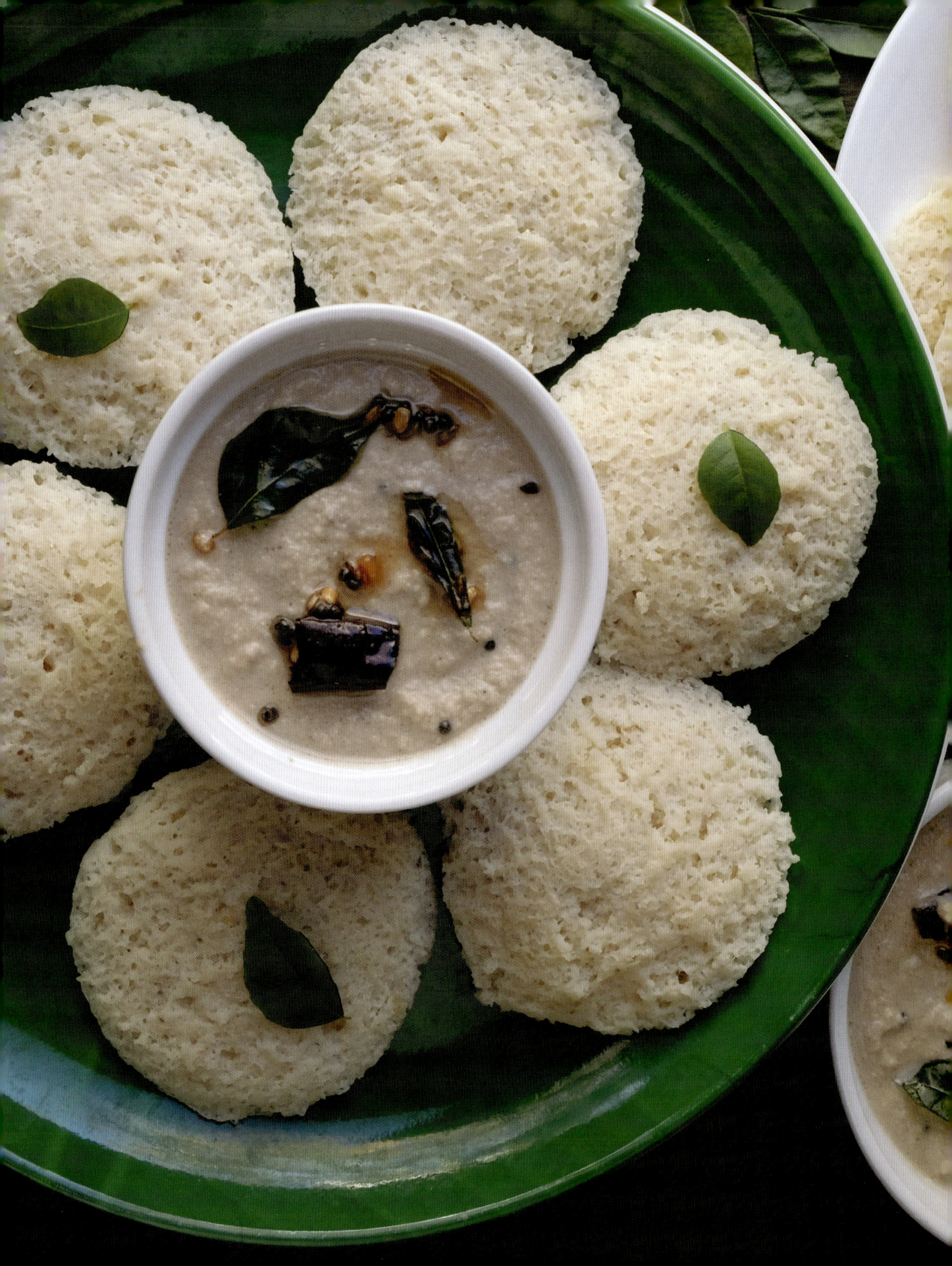

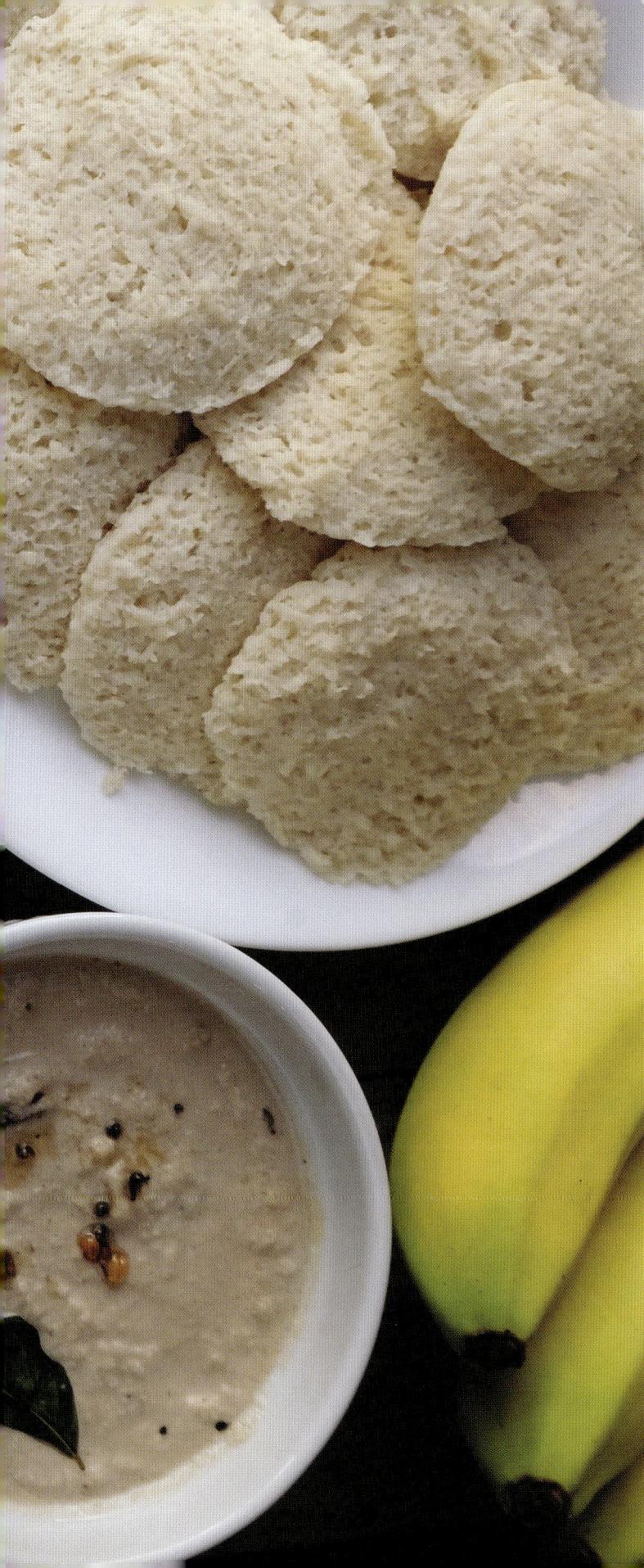

SCRUMPTIOUS BREAKFASTS

Whole Green Gram Dosa with Ginger Chutney	24
Sorghum (Jowar) Upma with Mint chutney	26
Upma without Rava with Peanut Chutney	27
Idlis Without Any Type of Rava with Coconut and Roasted Chickpea Dal Chutney	29
Finger Millet (Ragi) Idli with Sambar	30
Finger Millet (Ragi) and Black Gram (Urad Dal) Dosa with Tomato Chutney	31
Sorghum (Jowar) Idli with Green Chili Chutney	32
Finger Millet (Ragi) Upma with Curry Leaf Chutney	33
Buttermilk Steel Cut Oats	34
Multi-Millet Mini Idlis with Vegetable Broth	35

Idlis without any type of Rava with
Coconut and Roasted Chickpea Dal Chutney

WHOLE GREEN GRAM DOSA

The glycemic index of green gram is very low (38), and it contains a comparatively low amount of carbohydrates so the green gram dosa breakfast is highly recommended for Type 2 diabetics.

Ingredients

Whole green gram: 12 oz. (320 ml)

Green chilis: 6

Onion: 1, chopped

Ginger: 1 big piece, chopped

Cumin seeds: ½ teaspoon

Oil: sufficient quantity

Salt: sufficient quantity

Directions

Wash the green gram in water thoroughly and soak it in water for 12 hours. Then grind it, adding salt and a good amount of water to make it into a thin batter.

Heat a dosa (crêpe) pan, place some batter in it and spread it evenly to make a dosa (thin pancake). Put pieces of green chilis, onion, ginger and cumin seeds all over the dosa. Pour a small amount of oil all around the dosa, and a little amount of oil on the dosa itself. It is advisable to fry the dosa to a medium roast to preserve its flavor.

Ginger chutney is usually suggested for green gram dosa.

· ·

GINGER CHUTNEY

Ginger chutney has vitamin C, fiber, and antioxidants in good quantities to strengthen the immune system while making a tasty side dish.

Ingredients

Ginger: 1 large piece, cut into small pieces

Oil: 2 tablespoons

Black gram: 1 tablespoon

Fenugreek seeds: ⅓ teaspoon

Cumin: ⅓ teaspoon

Dry red chilis: 5

Tamarind juice: 6 oz. (160 ml)

Jaggery: 1 sufficiently large piece

Salt: sufficient quantity

Directions

Cut the ginger into small pieces, fry them in 1 tablespoon of oil and set them aside.

Then roast the black gram, fenugreek seeds, cumin, and dry red chilis in 1 tablespoon of oil. Mix in the roasted ginger.

Grind the mixture along with tamarind, jaggery, and salt, adding a small quantity of water as the ginger chutney, suitable for green gram dosa, has to be semi-thick. No garnishing is usually needed for it.

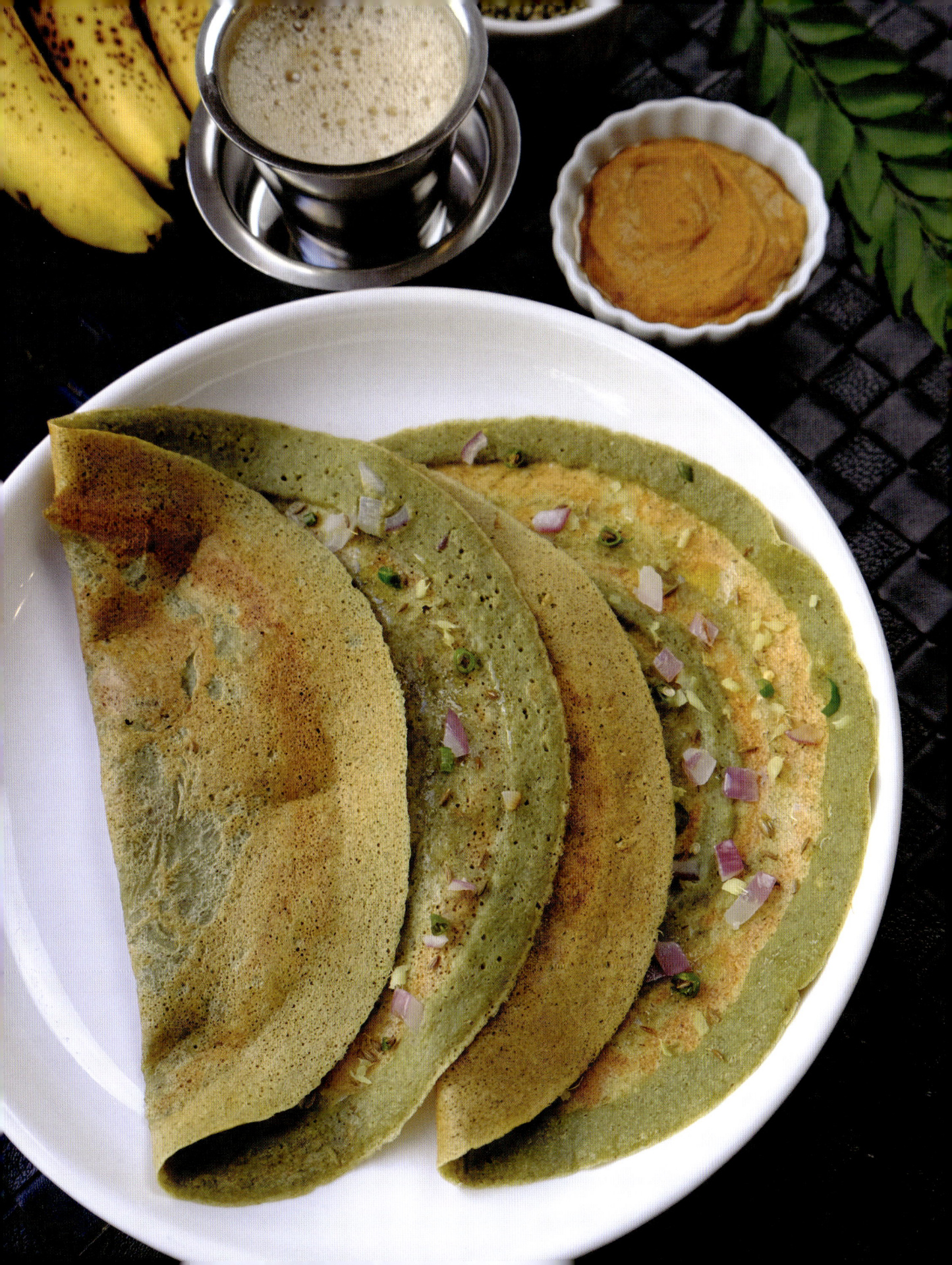

SORGHUM (JOWAR) UPMA

Ingredients

Jowar rava: 6 oz. (160 ml)

Oil: 2 tablespoons

Chickpea dal: ½ teaspoon

Black gram: ½ teaspoon

Mustard seeds: ¼ teaspoon

Cumin seeds: ¼ teaspoon

Green chilis: 3

Ginger: 1 small piece, diced

Onions: 1, chopped

Tomatoes: 1, chopped

Curry leaves: 2 stalks

Salt: sufficient quantity

Directions

Soak the jowar the whole night. Pour oil in a saucepan, and fry the chickpea dal, black gram, mustard seeds, and cumin seeds till soft. Then add the green chilis, ginger pieces, onion pieces, tomato pieces, salt and curry leaves to the above roasted ingredients, and keep them on a low flame for two minutes.

Add 18 oz. (480 ml) of water and boil for 10 minutes. Now add the sieved jowar rava to it and cook it for 30 minutes on a medium to a low flame, mixing it with a spoon. Add more water if required, until the jowar upma is ready.

Serve with the mint chutney recipe below.

. . . .

MINT CHUTNEY

Mint contains good amounts of vitamin C, fiber and antioxidants. Similarly, jowar has a low glycemic index, so white jowar upma with mint chutney keeps Type 2 diabetics healthy, besides controlling your blood sugar levels.

Ingredients

Mint leaves: 6 oz. (160 ml)

White sesame seeds: 1.5 oz. (40 ml)

Oil: 2 tablespoons

Dry red chilis: 6

Tomatoes: 1, chopped

Tamarind: sufficient quantity

Garlic: 5 cloves (optional)

Salt: sufficient quantity

Tempering ingredients

Black gram: ⅓ teaspoon • Dry red chilis: 1

Mustard seeds: ⅛ teaspoon

Curry leaves: 2 stalks • Asafetida: 1 pinch

Oil: 2 tablespoons • Cumin seeds: ⅛ teaspoon

Directions

Wash the mint leaves and dry them.

In a saucepan, roast the sesame seeds, then grind them and set the powder aside.

Then roast the mint leaves and chilis in a tablespoon of oil and set them aside.

Lightly fry the tomato pieces, garlic, and tamarind in a tablespoon of oil. Grind all the ingredients together in a mixie, adding sufficient water to your desired thickness and salt to taste.

Temper the chutney with the tempering ingredients after roasting them in oil.

UPMA WITHOUT RAVA

Upma rava contains a large quantity of carbohydrates and its glycemic index is also high (66), thus it spikes blood sugar levels. So here is an upma without rava, as tasty as the usual upma, but one that helps you keep your blood sugar in control while making you enjoy a yummy breakfast.

Ingredients

Cauliflower rice: 18 oz. (480 ml)

Oil: 2 tablespoons

Chickpea dal: 1 teaspoon

Black gram: 1 teaspoon

Mustard seeds: ¼ teaspoon

Cumin seeds: ¼ teaspoon

Asafetida: a pinch

Green chilis: 4

Ginger: 1 large piece cut into small ones

Onion: 1, chopped

Carrot: 1, chopped

Capsicum: 1

Tomatoes: 2, chopped

Coriander leaves: sufficient amount

Curry leaves: 2 stalks

Salt: sufficient quantity

Preparation of cauliflower rice

The cauliflower should be separated into florets and soaked in lukewarm water for 15 minutes. Allow them to dry for some time. Then grate them on a grater to produce cauliflower rice.

Directions for making upma

Heat the oil in a saucepan and put in the chickpea dal, black gram dal, mustard seeds, cumin seeds, and asafetida, and roast them. Add the green chilis, ginger cut into pieces, and onion pieces, and fry them for a short time till tender.

Add the carrot, capsicum, tomato, coriander, and curry leaves to the above mixture and fry them a little longer.

Put a lid on the saucepan and cook for 5 minutes.

Add the cauliflower rice and salt, then put the lid back. Cook on a low flame for 15 minutes. No water is needed as cauliflower rice has moisture in it. Serve when ready.

The suggested side dish is peanut chutney.

PEANUT CHUTNEY

Ingredients

Peanuts: 6 oz. (160 ml)

Green chilis: 6

Oil: 1 teaspoon

Tamarind juice: 1.5 oz. (40 ml)

Salt: sufficient quantity

Tempering ingredients

Oil: 1 tablespoon • Mustard seeds: $^1/_8$ teaspoon

Black gram: $^1/_3$ teaspoon • Asafetida: a pinch

Dry red chilis: 1 cut up • Curry leaves: 2 stalks

Directions

Fry the peanuts and green chilis together in a little oil in a saucepan or small frying pan. Then grind them along with tamarind juice and salt to a thin smooth paste, adding sufficient water.

Temper the chutney with the tempering ingredients after roasting them in oil. The upma with this yummy peanut chutney makes for an enjoyable breakfast.

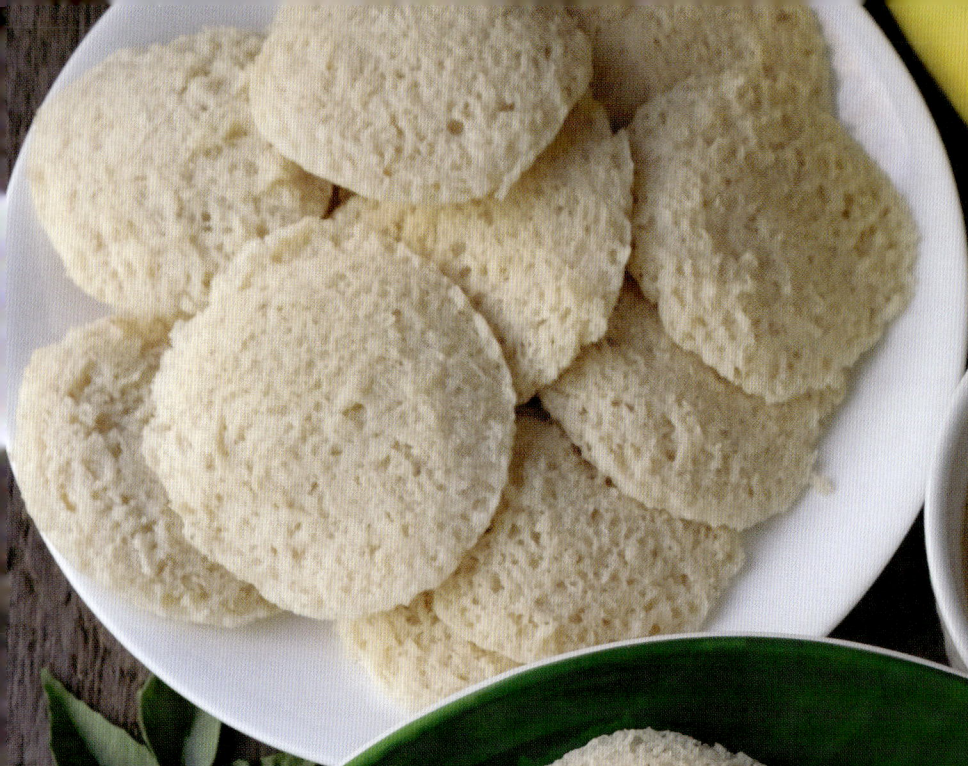

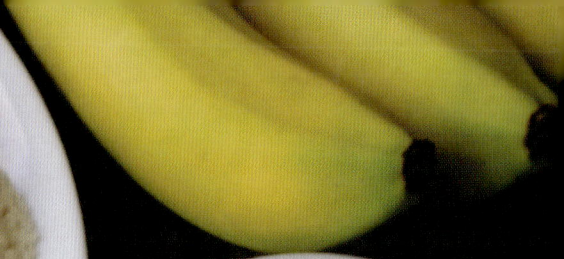

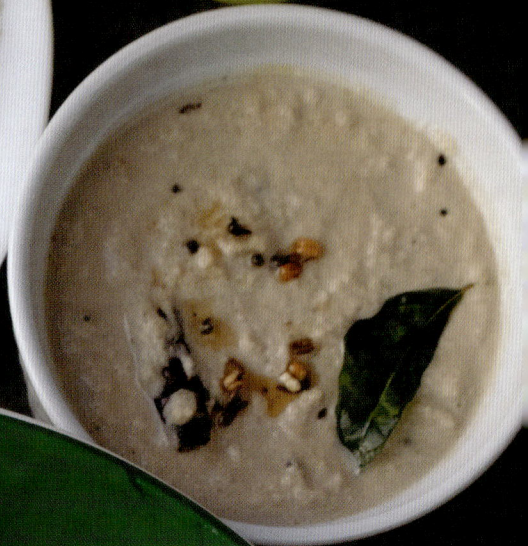

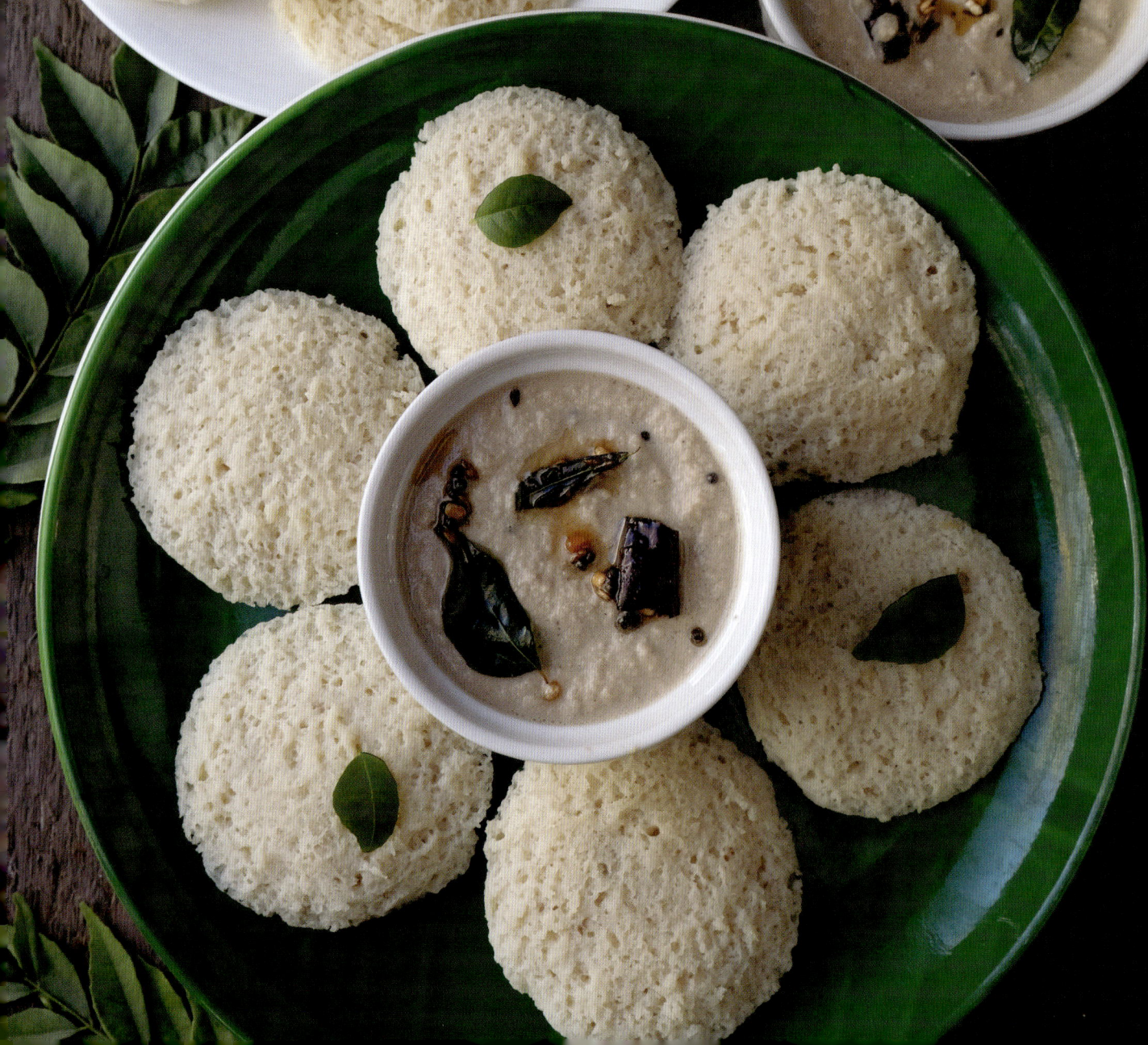

IDLIS WITHOUT ANY TYPE OF RAVA

We usually eat rava made from rice, millets, or jowar. Whatever the rava, it contains carbohydrates in some quantity. The following is thus a recipe for idlis without rava to make it more diabetes friendly. Since black gram and green gram have a very low glycemic index, these idlis will keep your blood sugar levels in control.

Ingredients

Black gram husked (urad dal): 6 oz. (160 ml)

Green gram husked (moong dal): 6 oz. (160 ml)

Fenugreek seeds: $1/3$ teaspoon

Salt: sufficient quantity

Directions

Soak the black gram and green gram along with fenugreek seeds for 6 hours. Then grind them together to a smooth batter of idli consistency. Add salt to the batter to taste and allow it to ferment for 10 hours. Then cook the batter in an idli cooker to make idlis, which will be as tasty as the usual version.

The suggested chutney is coconut and roasted chickpea chutney.

· ·

COCONUT AND ROASTED CHICKPEA DAL CHUTNEY

Urad dal, moong dal and chickpeas have low glycemic index and only a small amount of carbohydrates, plus many proteins and nutrients. So, this breakfast is highly recommended for people with Type 2 diabetes.

Ingredients

Green chilis: 6

Grated coconut: 6 oz. (160 ml)

Roasted chickpea dal: 6 oz. (160 ml)

Tamarind: a lemon sized piece

Salt: sufficient quantity

Tempering ingredients

Oil: 1 tablespoon

Dry red chilis: 1

Mustard seeds: $1/8$ teaspoon

Cumin seeds: $1/8$ teaspoon

Black gram: $1/3$ teaspoon

Asafetida: a pinch

Curry leaves: 2 stalks

Directions

Fry the green chilis partially in oil in a small saucepan or frying pan. Then grind the grated coconut, roasted chickpeas, tamarind, salt and the green chilis with a sufficient quantity of water.

Next, roast the tempering ingredients together in oil in a small frying pan. Add the roasted ingredients to the chutney and eat with the idlis not only for enjoyment but also to get control over your Type 2 diabetes.

FINGER MILLET (RAGI) IDLI

Finger millet has a comparatively low glycemic index when cooked. It has a good fiber content, so it helps keep blood sugar levels in control. Taken with sambar, finger millet idlis are a yummy breakfast.

Ingredients

Black gram (husked):6 oz. (160 ml)
Finger millet rava: 18 oz. (480 ml)
Fenugreek: ½ teaspoon
Salt: sufficient quantity

Directions

Soak the black gram and fenugreek for 10 hours, then grind them.

Mix the finger millet rava in it, adding salt and water as needed. The batter should be of idli consistency. Allow it to ferment for 12 hours.

Cook the idlis in an idli cooker. Eaten with sambar, they make a delicious meal.

. . . .

SAMBAR

Ingredients

Pigeon pea (toor dal): 4.5 oz (120 ml)
Tamarind juice: 12 oz. (320 ml)
Onions: 2, chopped
Green chilis: 2, chopped
Bottle gourd: ¼ piece
Curry leaves: 2 stalks, chopped
Coriander leaves: 3 oz.
(80 ml), chopped
Sambar powder: 3 to 4 teaspoons
Turmeric powder: ¼ teaspoon
Jaggery: small to medium piece
Salt: sufficient quantity
Chickpea flour: 1 teaspoon

Tempering ingredients

Oil: 1 tablespoon
Dry red chilis: 2
Mustard seeds: ¼ teaspoon
Asafetida: a pinch
Cumin seeds: ¼ teaspoon
Curry leaves: 1 stalk

Directions

Cook the pigeon pea in a pressure cooker. Then in a saucepan, mix the softly cooked dal with tamarind juice, and add all the vegetables after cutting them into pieces, including green chilis, curry leaves and coriander leaves as well as sambar powder, salt, turmeric powder and jaggery. Cook all of this in a sufficient volume of water. It takes 20 minutes for the sambar to cook on a medium flame.

After the sambar has cooked well, temper it with all the tempering ingredients after roasting them in oil in a small frying pan.

Add one teaspoon of chickpea flour mixed in a small cup of water to the sambar to improve the consistency.

FINGER MILLET (RAGI) AND BLACK GRAM (URAD DAL) DOSA

Black gram has a very low glycemic index. Ragi also has a comparatively low glycemic index besides being rich in fiber. So ragi and black gram dosas are a diabetes-friendly food. Taken with the mouth-watering tomato chutney, these dosas will be a culinary delight.

Ingredients

Finger millet: 12 oz. (320 ml)

Black gram (husked): 3 oz. (80 ml)

Fenugreek seeds: ½ teaspoon

Flattened rice: 1.5 oz. (40 ml)

Salt: sufficient amount

Directions

Soak the finger millet for 12 hours, black gram and fenugreek for 6 hours, and flattened rice for 10 minutes.

Grind them together into a smooth batter, mixing in some salt. Allow the batter to ferment for 12 hours. The consistency has to be thin.

Using a little oil, roast the dosas on both sides on a dosa pan. I suggest tomato chutney for these dosas.

TOMATO CHUTNEY

Ingredients

White sesame seeds: 1.5 oz. (40 ml) (optional)

Tomatoes: 3 or 4

Green chilis: 5 or 6

Dry red chilis: 3

Tamarind: sufficient quantity

Salt: sufficient quantity

Oil: 1 tablespoon

Tempering ingredients

Mustard seeds: ¼ teaspoon

Cumin seeds: ¼ teaspoon

Curry leaves: 2 stalks

Black gram: ½ teaspoon

Asafetida: one pinch

Oil: 1 tablespoon

Directions

Roast the white sesame seeds and grind them into a powder.

Grind the tomatoes, green chilis, and red chilis after roasting them in oil, along with tamarind and salt in a sufficient quantity of water.

Mix the sesame powder in.

Temper the chutney with the tempering ingredients after sufficiently roasting them in oil.

SORGHUM (JOWAR) IDLI

Sorghum has a low glycemic index and is rich in fiber and antioxidants besides being gluten free. It makes good food for Type 2 diabetics.

Ingredients

Sorghum rava: 12 oz. (320 ml)

Black gram (husked): 6 oz. (160 ml)

Fenugreek: ½ teaspoon

Idli rava: 1.5 oz. (40 ml)

Salt: sufficient quantity

Directions

Soak the sorghum rava for 12 hours, and soak the black gram and fenugreek for 6 hours.

Grind the black gram and fenugreek to a smooth batter.

Mix the sorghum rava and idli rava in the black gram batter and allow it to ferment for about 10 hours.

Mix in salt and make idlis in an idli cooker.

The suggested chutney to accompany this is green chili chutney.

GREEN CHILI CHUTNEY

Ingredients

Black gram: 2 teaspoons

Coriander seeds: 1 teaspoon

Cumin seeds: ⅓ teaspoon

Green chilis: 150 grams (⅓ lb.)

Oil: 2 tablespoons

Coriander leaves: ½ bunch

Garlic: 6 cloves (optional)

Tamarind juice: 6 oz.
(160 ml)

Salt: sufficient quantity

Jaggery: a medium sized piece

Directions

Fry the black gram, coriander seeds, and cumin seeds without using oil. Grind the mixture and set the powder aside.

Then lightly fry green chilis in two tablespoons of oil and keep them on the stove for 5 minutes, putting a lid on the frying pan to keep it warm.

Grind the green chilis, coriander leaves, and garlic (optional) along with tamarind juice and salt into a paste. Mix the black gram, coriander, and cumin powder into the paste and grind them together a little. Tempering is not necessary, but if you want, you can temper the mixture with mustard seeds, black gram, asafetida, and curry leaves after roasting them in oil.

FINGER MILLET (RAGI) UPMA

Ragi has a low glycemic index, supplemented with its rich fiber content to keep blood sugar levels in check. Curry leaves are rich in antioxidants and improve digestion. So, ragi upma with curry leaf chutney is highly beneficial.

Ingredients

Finger millet rava: 6 oz. (160 ml)

Bombay rava (suji): 3 oz. (80 ml)

Oil: 2 tablespoons

Mustard seeds: ¼ teaspoon

Cumin seeds: ¼ teaspoon

Dry red chilis: 1

Cashew nuts: 8 (optional)

Black gram: ½ teaspoon

Chickpea dal: ½ teaspoon

Ginger: 1 small piece

Onion: 1, chopped

Green chilis: 4

Tomatoes: 12 oz. (320 ml), chopped

Curry leaves: 2 stalks

Ghee: 2 tablespoons

Coriander leaves: 4 stems

Directions

First roast the Bombay rava sufficiently and set it aside.

Heat oil in a saucepan and add the mustard seeds, cumin, dry red chili pieces, cashews, black gram, and chickpea dal. Roast them well. Add the ginger, onion, and green chili pieces to the above roasted items and fry them a little. Add the tomatoes and curry leaves and roast them a little more.

Put a lid on the saucepan and allow all the above ingredients to cook for 5 minutes. Add the Bombay rava, finger millet rava, and salt to the roasted and cooked vegetables.

Add 24 oz. (640 ml) of boiling water to the above mix. Stir the rava with a spoon to prevent lumps. Keep the saucepan on a low to medium flame for 20 minutes.

Garnish with coriander leaves and (if desired) cashew nuts roasted in ghee. This yummy ragi upma is ready for your enjoyment.

A good side dish is curry leaf chutney.

CURRY LEAF CHUTNEY

Ingredients

Curry leaves: 30 oz. (800 ml)

Dry red chilis: 6

Black gram: 1 teaspoon

Oil: 1 tablespoon

Tamarind: sufficient quantity

Garlic: 3 cloves (optional)

Cumin powder: ½ teaspoon

Jaggery: a small piece

Salt: sufficient quantity

Directions

Fry the curry leaves, dry red chilis, and black gram in oil. Then add the garlic (optional) along with cumin powder.

After the mixture becomes cool, add the tamarind, jaggery and salt, and grind it, adding sufficient water to get your desired consistency. The chutney has to be neither too thick nor too thin.

Temper the chutney with the tempering ingredients after frying them in oil.

Tempering ingredients

Mustard seeds: ⅛ teaspoon • Oil: 2 teaspoons

Black gram: ⅓ teaspoon • Asafetida: a pinch

BUTTERMILK STEEL CUT OATS

This steel cut oat preparation makes not only a diabetes-friendly food in view of its low glycemic index, fiber content, and antioxidant properties, but also a very tasty breakfast.

Ingredients

Steel cut oats: 12 oz. (320 ml)
Buttermilk: 18 oz. (480 ml)
Coriander leaves: 1.5 oz. (40 ml), chopped
Green chilis: 2
Cumin seeds: 1/8 teaspoon
Salt: sufficient quantity

Directions

Boil the steel cut oats in 24 oz. (640 ml) of water for 1 hour on a low flame. Allow the oats to cool.

Mix in the buttermilk.

Grind coriander leaves and green chilis into a paste. Add the paste along with salt and cumin seeds to the oats. Serve and enjoy.

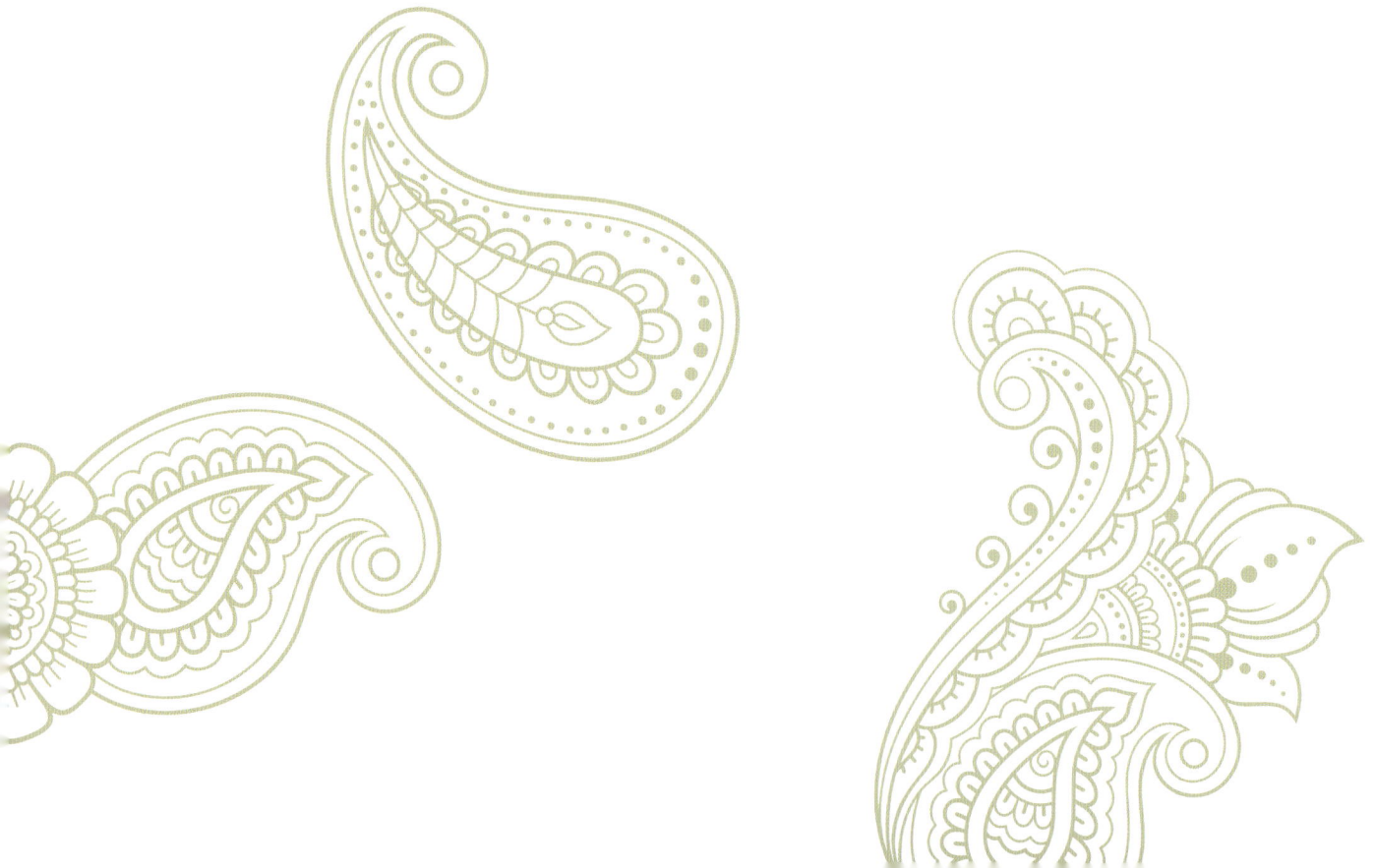

MULTI-MILLET MINI IDLIS

Black gram, ragi, foxtail millet and horse gram all have a low glycemic index and contain good amounts of nutrients. These idlis are highly recommended for Type 2 diabetics. Along with the vegetable broth, multi-millet idlis provide a delicious breakfast.

Ingredients

Black gram (husked): 3 oz. (80 ml)

Finger millet (ragi): 1.5 oz. (40 ml)

Foxtail millet: 1.5 oz. (40 ml)

Horse gram: 1.5 oz. (40 ml)

Fenugreek seeds: ½ teaspoon

Salt: sufficient quantity

Directions

Soak the black gram, ragi, foxtail millet, horse gram, and fenugreek seeds for 12 hours. Then grind them into a smooth batter. Allow the batter to ferment for 12 hours. Add salt to the batter as desired.

Cook mini idlis in a mini idli cooker.

The suggested side dish is a delicious vegetable broth.

VEGETABLE BROTH

Ingredients

Bottle gourd pieces: 18 oz. (480 ml)

Brinjal pieces: 6 oz. (160 ml)

Carrot pieces: 6 oz. (160 ml)

Onion pieces: 6 oz. (160 ml)

Tamarind juice: 9 oz. (240 ml)

Green chilis: 2, cut into pieces

Coriander: ¼ bunch

Curry leaves: 2 stalks

Salt: sufficient quantity

Jaggery: a small to medium piece

Turmeric powder: a small quantity

Tempering ingredients

Oil: 1 tablespoon

Mustard seeds: $1/8$ teaspoon

Cumin seeds: $1/8$ teaspoon

Dry red chilis: 1

Asafetida: a pinch

Curry leaves: 2 stalks

Garlic: 2 cloves (optional)

Directions

Put all the cut vegetables in the tamarind juice in a saucepan. Add the green chilis, and coriander leaves. Add salt, jaggery, and turmeric powder. Boil the broth until all the vegetables are sufficiently cooked.

Roast the tempering ingredients in oil in a small frying pan. Add garlic (optional) during the final stages of frying. Add the tempering mixture to the broth. Serve and enjoy.

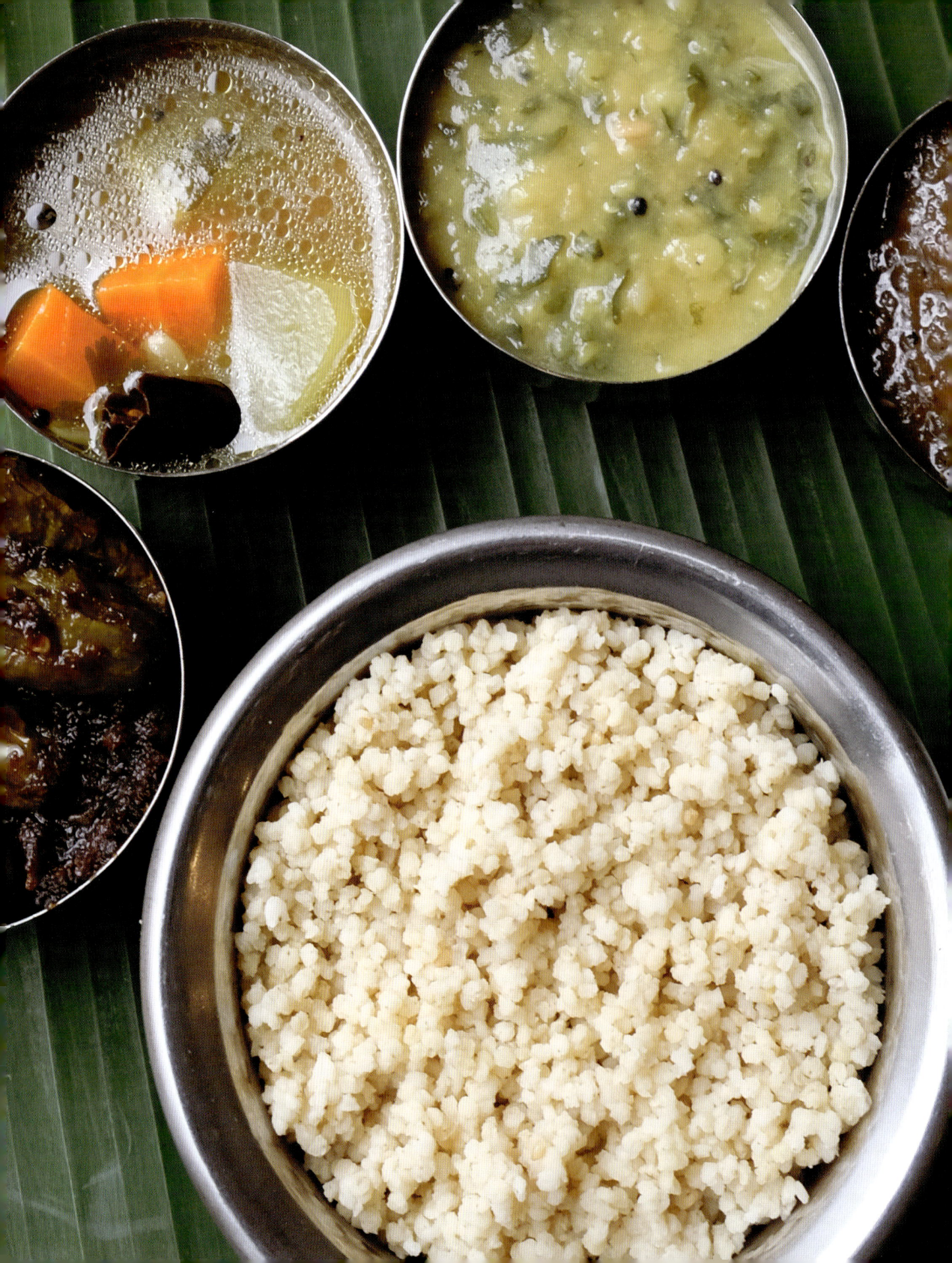

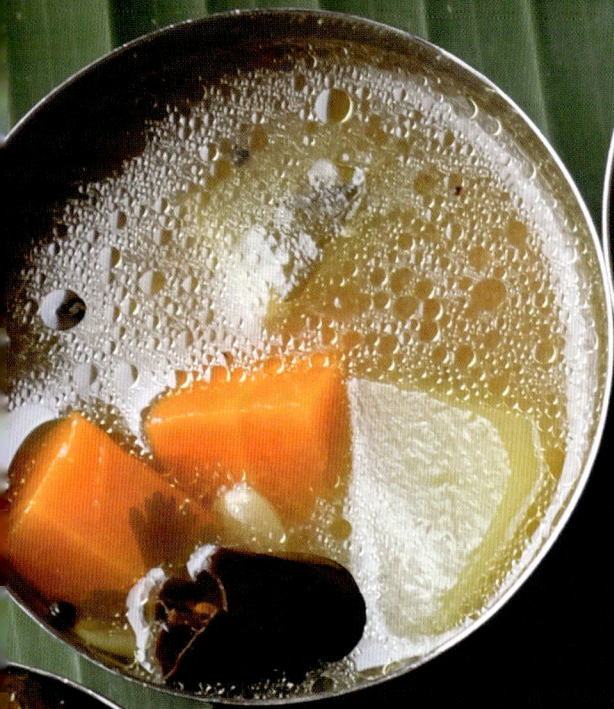

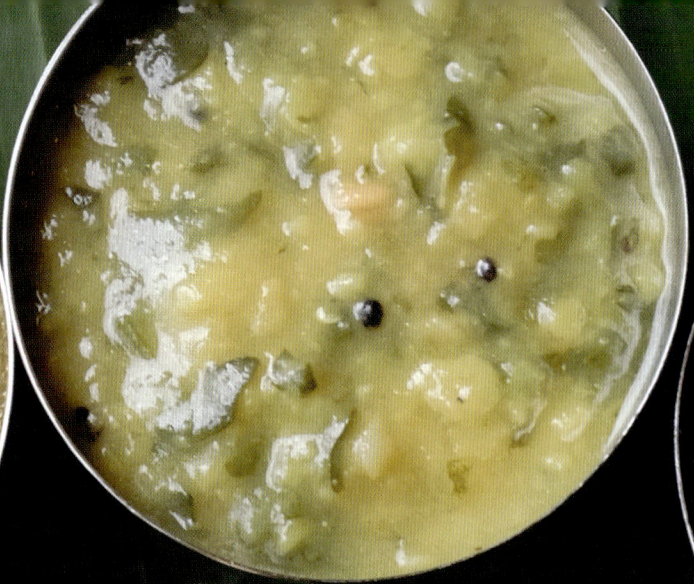

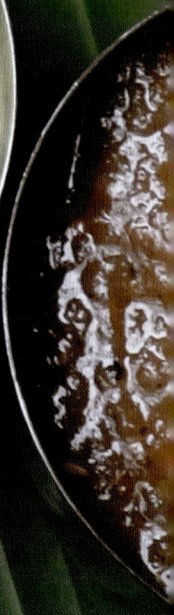

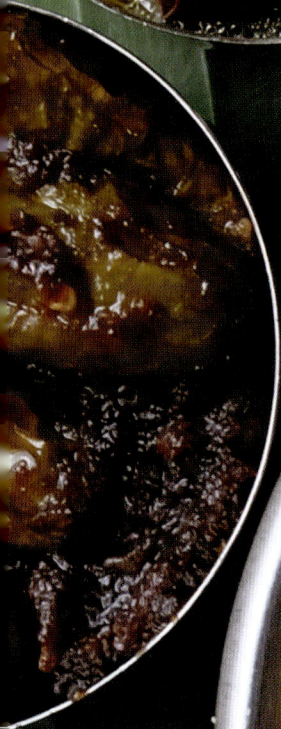

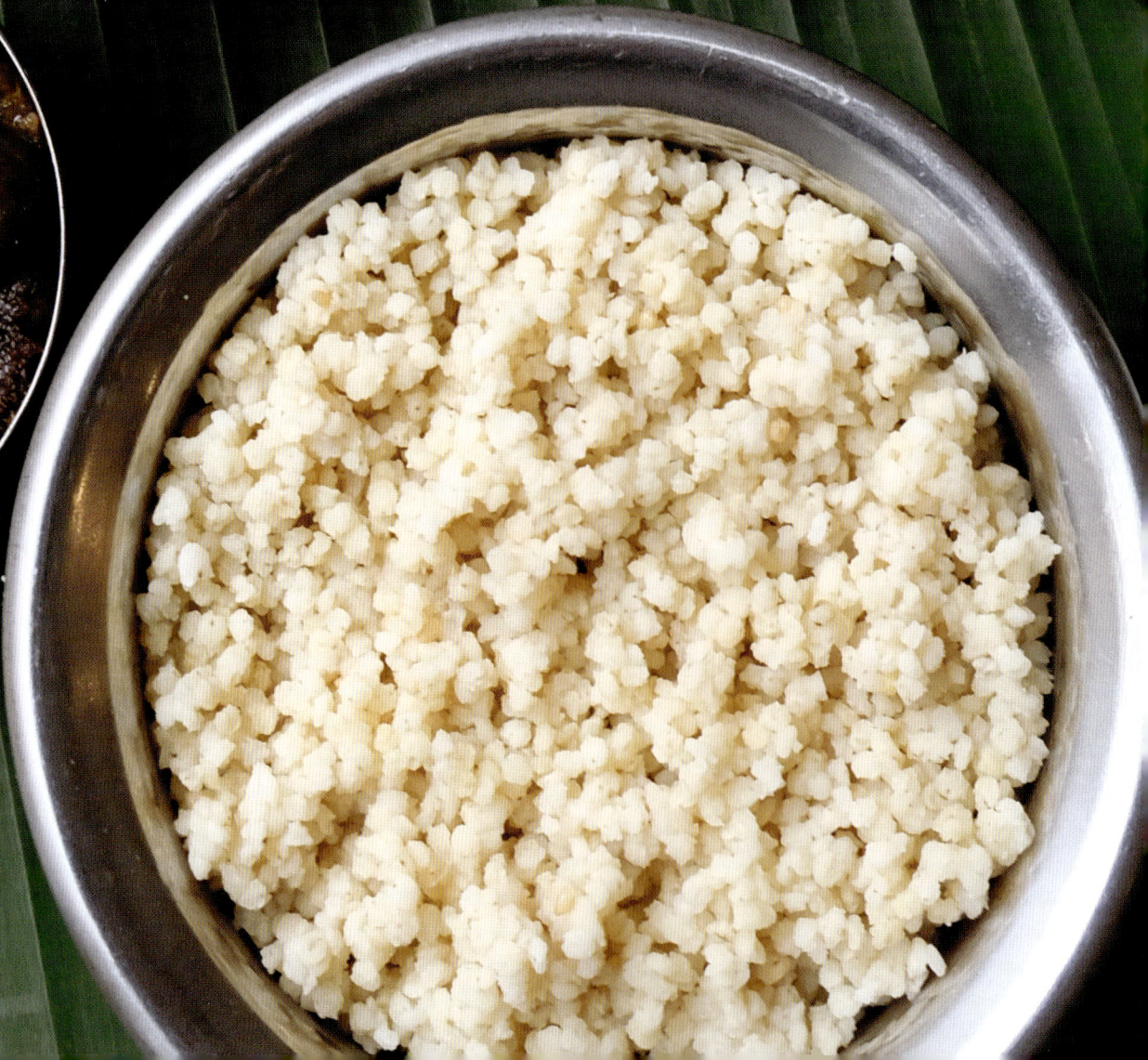

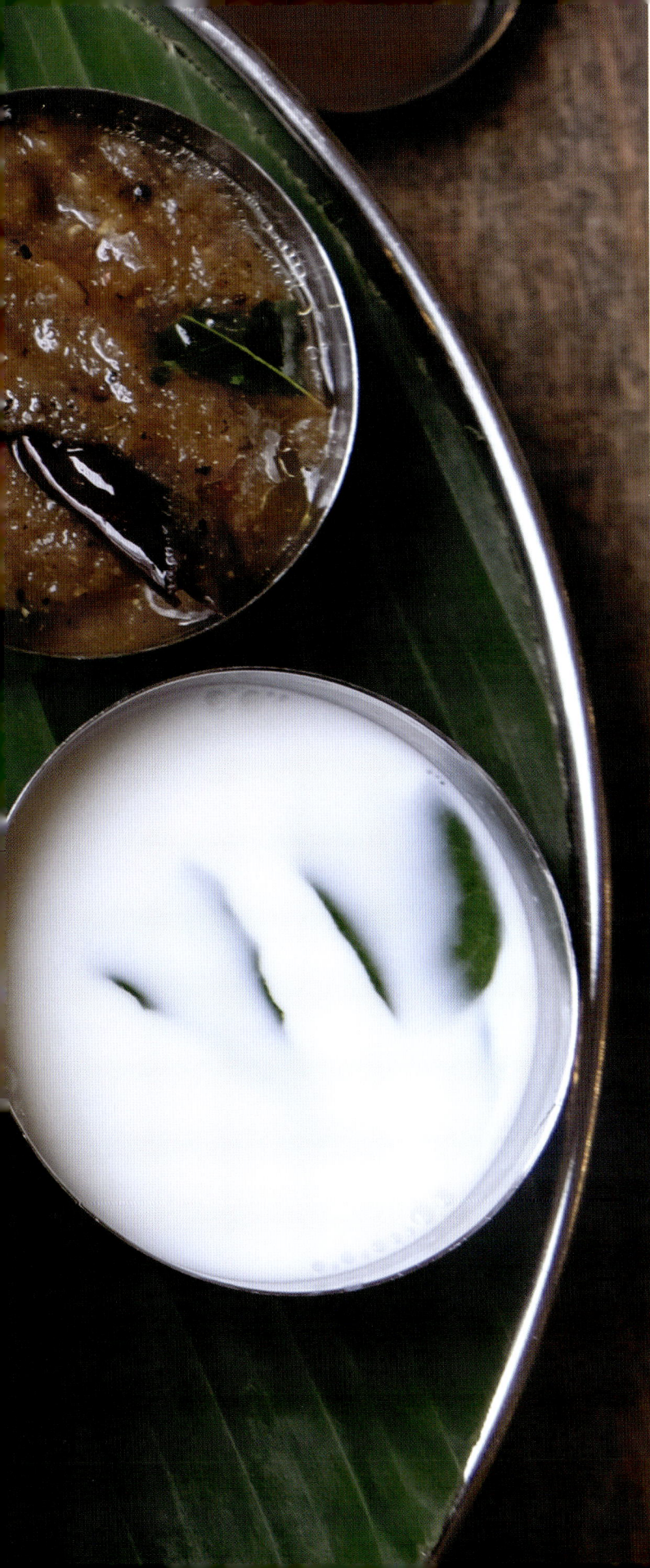

MULTI-COURSE LUNCHES

Foxtail Millet Lunch: Cooked Foxtail Millet, Fenugreek Leaf Dal, Tindora Curry with Onion Paste, Yellow Cucumber Chutney, Mixed Vegetable Stew, Buttermilk

PEARL MILLET LUNCH
Cooked Pearl Millet • Sorrel Leaf Dal • Bitter Gourd Fry • Coriander Chutney • Onion Stew • Buttermilk (optional)

COOKED PEARL MILLET

Pearl millet has a lower glycemic index and less carbohydrate content besides many good properties. So, it is a good choice for people with diabetes.

Ingredients
Pearl millet: 6 oz. (160 ml)

Directions
Soak the pearl millet for 12 hours and cook it in a pressure cooker with 18 oz. (480 ml) of water.

· ·

SORREL LEAF DAL

Ingredients
Pigeon pea (toor dal): 2 oz. (50 ml)
Sorrel leaves: ½ bunch (about 24 oz.)
Garlic: 4 cloves (optional)
Green chilis: 2
Turmeric: a pinch
Salt: sufficient quantity

Tempering ingredients
Mustard seeds: ⅛ teaspoon
Cumin seeds: ⅓ teaspoon
Dry red chilis: 1
Curry leaves: 2 stalks
Asafetida: a pinch
Oil: 1 tablespoon

Directions
Cook the pigeon pea and sorrel leaves along with the garlic cloves (optional), green chilis, and turmeric in a good amount of water to bring it to a semi-thick consistency.

After it is fully cooked, add salt. Depending on the sourness of the sorrel, you can adjust the number of green chilis.

Temper the dal with the tempering ingredients after frying them.

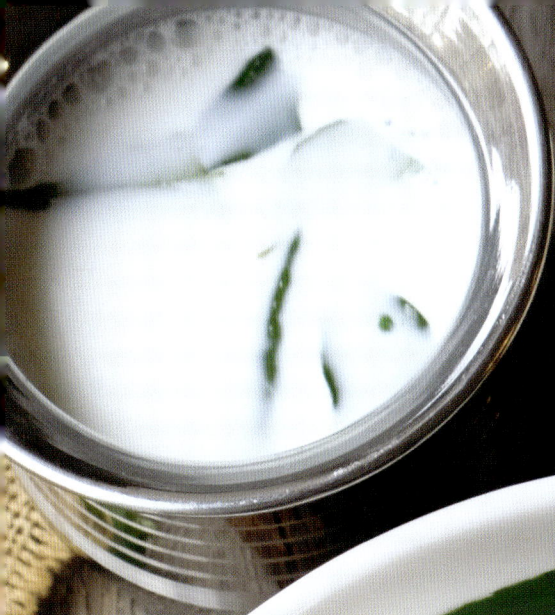

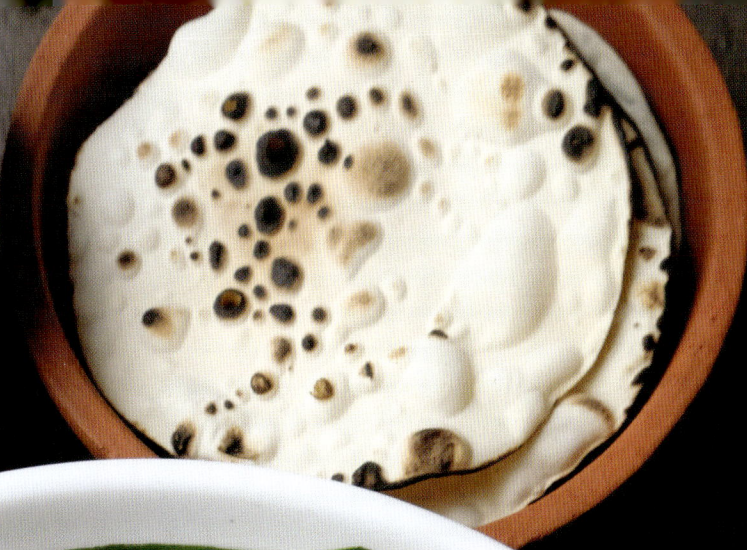

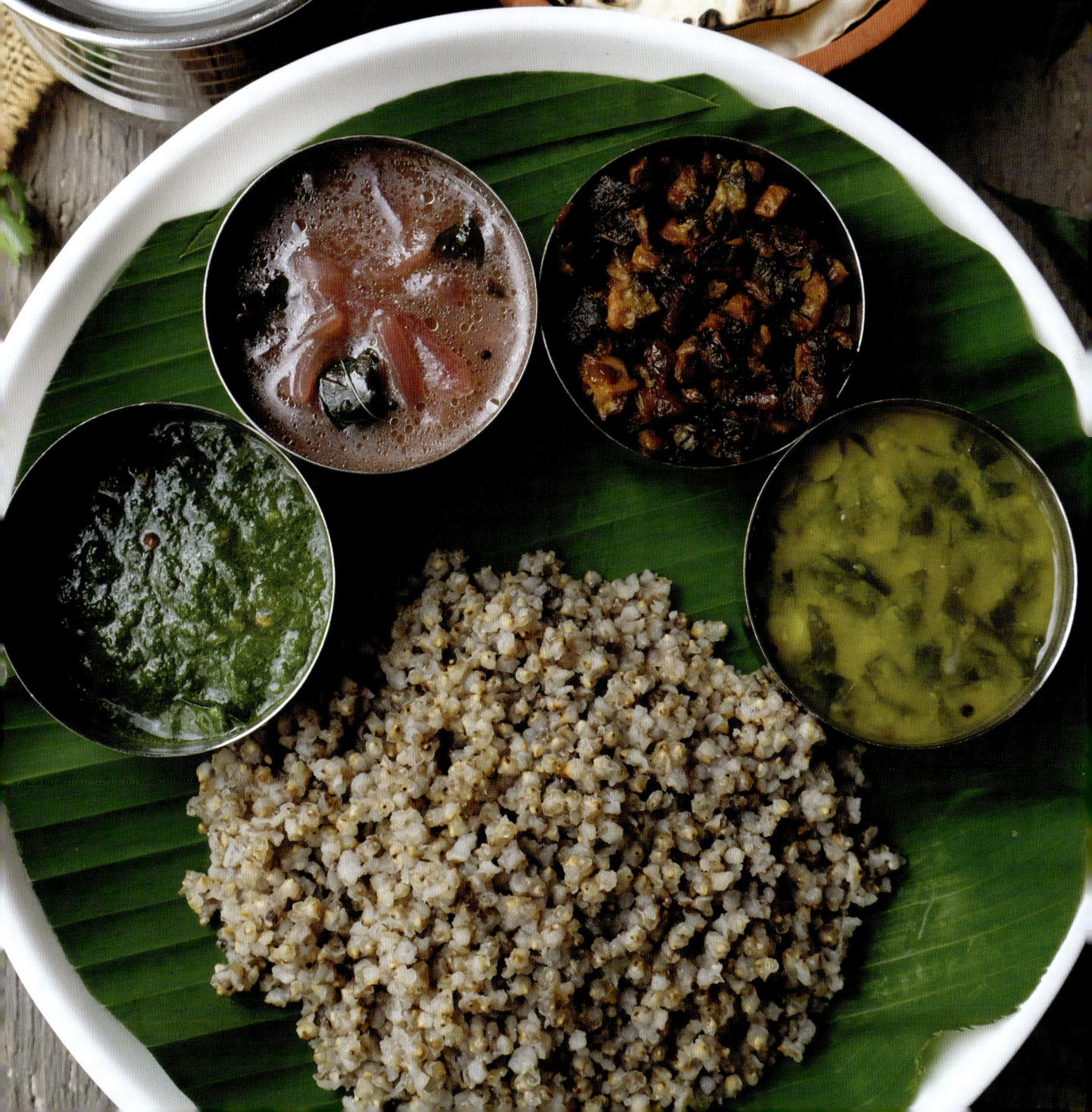

BITTER GOURD FRY

Ingredients

Bitter gourds: 4, cut into pieces
Onions: 2, cut into pieces
Oil: 3 tablespoons
Tamarind juice: a small quantity
Red chili cumin powder: ½ teaspoon
Salt: sufficient quantity

Directions

Cut the bitter gourds and onions into pieces.

Fry the bitter gourd in oil. After it is fried to some extent, add tamarind juice and onions, and fry them further. Close the saucepan with a lid to use less oil. (You can leave out the tamarind juice depending on your taste. Tamarind juice reduces the degree of the bitterness of bitter gourd.)

Once it is fully fried and cooked, add the dry red chili cumin powder and salt to taste.

CORIANDER CHUTNEY

Ingredients

Coriander leaves: 1 bunch
Green chilis: 5
Tamarind juice: 2 oz. (50 ml)
Jaggery: a medium sized piece
Garlic: 3 cloves (optional)
Salt: sufficient quantity

Tempering ingredients

Mustard seeds: ¹/₈ teaspoon
Black gram: ¹/₃ teaspoon
Asafetida: a pinch
Curry leaves: 2 stalks
Dry red chilis: 1, cut into pieces
Oil: 2 tablespoons

Directions

Wash the coriander leaves thoroughly, then grind them with the green chilis, tamarind, jaggery, garlic cloves (optional), and salt into a smooth paste.

Temper the chutney with the tempering ingredients after roasting them in oil.

ONION STEW

Ingredients

Onions sliced: 18 oz. (480 ml)

Green chilis: 1, split into halves

Coriander leaves: a small quantity, chopped

Tamarind juice: 6 oz. (160 ml)

Turmeric: 1 pinch

Salt: sufficient quantity

Jaggery: a small quantity

Chickpea flour: ½ teaspoon

Tempering ingredients

Mustard seeds: ⅛ teaspoon

Dry red chilis: 2, cut into pieces

Asafetida: 1 pinch

Curry leaves: 2 stalks

Oil: 1 tablespoon

Directions

Place the onions, green chili split into halves, chopped coriander leaves, turmeric, jaggery, tamarind juice, and salt in a saucepan. Cook the ingredients, adding sufficient volume of water, to arrive at a tasty stew.

Temper the stew with the tempering ingredients after roasting them in oil.

Mix the chickpea flour in the stew for good consistency and taste.

- -

BUTTERMILK MADE FROM YOGURT (OPTIONAL)

Ingredients

Curd (Yogurt): 6 oz (160ml)

Salt: sufficient quantity (optional)

Directions

Mix 12 oz. (320 ml) of water in curd (yogurt) to prepare the buttermilk. The yogurt can be unfermented or sour (fermented), depending on your taste.

LITTLE MILLET LUNCH

Cooked Little Millet • Drumstick Leaf Dal • Okra (Lady's Finger) Curry • Brinjal Chutney • Plain Rasam • Buttermilk (optional)

COOKED LITTLE MILLET

Little Millet has a low glycemic index besides being rich in fiber, nutrients, and minerals. It is highly recommended for Type 2 diabetics.

Ingredients

Little millet: 6 oz. (160 ml)

Directions

Wash the little millet in water and soak it for 12 hours.

Cook the millet in 14 oz. (360 ml) of water in a pressure cooker.

DRUMSTICK LEAF DAL

Ingredients

Green gram (moong dal) husked: 3 oz. (80 ml)
Drumstick leaves: 24 oz. (640 ml)
Salt: sufficient quantity

Tempering ingredients

Oil: 1 tablespoon
Mustard seeds: 1/8 teaspoon
Black gram: 1/3 teaspoon
Dry red chilis: 1
Curry leaves: 2 stalks
Asafetida: 1 pinch
Turmeric: 1 pinch

Directions

Wash the husked split green gram (moong dal) and drumstick leaves in water. Then cook them in a sufficient quantity of water in a saucepan to make the dal. Add salt after it has been cooked.

Temper the dal with the tempering ingredients after roasting them in oil.

OKRA (LADY'S FINGER) CURRY

Ingredients

Okras: 20, cut into pieces

Mustard seeds: ¼ teaspoon

Black gram: ½ teaspoon

Asafetida: 1 pinch

Dry red chilis: 2, cut into pieces

Curry leaves: 2 stalks

Oil: 1 tablespoon

Tamarind juice: sufficient quantity

Salt: sufficient quantity

Directions

Cut the okras into pieces.

Heat oil in a saucepan and add the mustard seeds, black gram (urad dal), asafetida, dry red chilis, and curry leaves, and roast them.

Add the tamarind juice and salt to the above roasted ingredients. Mix, then add the cut okra pieces. Cook the curry in a closed saucepan with a lid. No water is needed.

BRINJAL CHUTNEY

Ingredients

Brinjal: 1 large sized

Dry red chilis: 2

White sesame seeds: 2 teaspoons

Green chilis: 2

Salt: sufficient quantity

Tamarind: sufficient quantity

Garlic: 2 cloves (optional)

Coriander leaves: for garnishing

Tempering ingredients

Mustard seeds: $1/8$ teaspoon

Dry red chilis: 2, cut into pieces

Black gram: $1/3$ teaspoon

Asafetida: a pinch

Curry leaves: 2 stalks

Oil: 1 tablespoon

Directions

Take the brinjal and roast it over a flame after piercing it with a knife. After the brinjal cools down, peel it and extract the pulp.

Roast the dry red chilis with white sesame seeds, then grind them into a powder.

Add the brinjal pulp, green chilis, salt, tamarind, and garlic (optional) to the dry chili-sesame powder and grind it into a smooth chutney.

Temper the chutney with the tempering ingredients after roasting them in oil.

Garnish with coriander leaves and enjoy.

PLAIN RASAM

Ingredients

Black peppers: 12

Ginger: a small piece

Dry red chilis: 1

Tamarind: a small piece

Jaggery: a small piece

Salt: sufficient quantity

Turmeric: a pinch

Tempering ingredients

Mustard seeds: 1/8 teaspoon

Asafetida: 1 pinch

Cumin seeds: 1/8' teaspoon

Curry leaves: 2 stalks

Oil: 1 tablespoon

Directions

Grind the black pepper seeds, red chilis, and ginger into a paste.

In a saucepan, pour 24 oz. (640 ml) of water over the above mixture. Add the tamarind, jaggery, and salt. Boil it thoroughly.

Temper the rasam with the tempering ingredients after roasting them in oil.

· ·

BUTTERMILK MADE FROM YOGURT (OPTIONAL)

Ingredients

Curd (Yogurt): 6 oz (160ml)

Salt: sufficient quantity (optional)

Directions

Mix 12 oz. (320 ml) of water in curd (yogurt) to prepare the buttermilk. The yogurt can be unfermented or sour (fermented), depending on your taste.

KODO MILLET LUNCH

Cooked Kodo Millet • Amaranth Dal • Brinjal-Bean Curry • Mango-Coconut Chutney • Buttermilk Stew • Buttermilk (optional)

COOKED KODO MILLET

Kodo millet has a low glycemic index besides being rich in fiber, minerals and nutrients. It is highly recommended for Type 2 diabetics.

Ingredients

Kodo millet: 6 oz. (160 ml)

Directions

Wash the kodo millet in water and soak it for 12 hours. Drain, then add 12 oz. (320 ml) of fresh water to the soaked kodo millet and cook it in a pressure cooker.

. . . .

AMARANTH DAL

Ingredients

Pigeon pea (toor dal): 3 oz. (80 ml)

Amaranth leaves: 1 bunch

Salt: sufficient quantity

Tempering ingredients

Mustard seeds: ⅛ teaspoon

Dry red chilis: 2

Black gram: ⅛ teaspoon

Turmeric: 1 pinch

Asafetida: 1 pinch

Curry leaves: 2 stalks

Oil: 1 tablespoon

Directions

Wash the toor dal and amaranth leaves. Boil the toor dal and the amaranth together until soft.

Temper the amaranth dal with the tempering ingredients after roasting them in oil. Add salt to the amaranth dal.

BRINJAL-BEAN CURRY

Ingredients

Brinjals (eggplants): 6, chopped into pieces
Beans: 12 oz. (320 ml)
Salt: sufficient quantity
Ginger: 1 small piece
Green chilis: 2
Chickpea powder: 1 teaspoon

Tempering ingredients

Mustard seeds: 1/8 teaspoon
Chickpea dal: 1/3 teaspoon
Black gram dal: 1/3 teaspoon
Dry red chilis: 2
Asafetida: 1 pinch
Curry leaves: 2 stalks
Oil: 1 tablespoon

Directions

Wash the brinjals, then chop them into pieces. Cook the chopped brinjal and beans together in sufficient quantity of water. Add salt if needed.

Roast the tempering ingredients in oil in a frying pan.

Grind the ginger and green chilis into a paste and add it to the roasted tempering items. Roast it for one additional minute.

Add the roasted mixture to the cooked brinjal-bean. Close the lid and keep it on a flame for two minutes.

Mix the chickpea powder into the curry and keep it on a low flame for one minute. Your tasty brinjal-bean curry is now ready.

MANGO-COCONUT CHUTNEY

Ingredients

Dry red chilis: 5
Oil: 1 tablespoon
Green mango: 1, peeled and cut into pieces
Coconut: 12 oz. (320 ml), cut into pieces
Green chilis: 5
Salt: sufficient quantity

Tempering ingredients

Mustard seeds: 1/8 teaspoon
Black gram: 1/3 teaspoon
Dry red chilis: 1
Asafetida: 1 pinch
Curry leaves: 2 stalks
Turmeric powder: a little
Oil: 1 tablespoon

Directions

Roast the dry red chilis in oil.

Peel the green mango and cut it into small pieces. Grind the mango and coconut along with the roasted dry red chilis, green chilis, and salt.

Temper the chutney with the tempering ingredients after roasting them in oil. Serve and enjoy.

BUTTERMILK STEW

Ingredients

Buttermilk (thick and sour): 24 oz. (640 ml)

Chickpea flour: 1 tablespoon

Bottle gourd: ¼ piece

Green chilis: 1

Salt: sufficient quantity

Coriander leaves: a small quantity

Turmeric powder: a pinch

Tempering ingredients

Oil: 1 tablespoon

Mustard seeds: ⅛ teaspoon

Dry red chilis: 2

Asafetida: 1 pinch

Curry leaves: 2 stalks

Directions

Mix the chickpea flour into the buttermilk. Whisk to be sure that there are no lumps of flour in the buttermilk.

Pour the buttermilk into a saucepan and add the bottle gourd pieces, split green chili, salt, coriander leaves, and turmeric powder. Boil the mixture for 20 minutes.

Temper the stew with the tempering ingredients after roasting them in oil.

· ·

BUTTERMILK MADE FROM YOGURT (OPTIONAL)

Ingredients

Curd (Yogurt): 6 oz (160ml)

Salt: sufficient quantity (optional)

Directions

Mix 12 oz. (320 ml) of water in curd (yogurt) to prepare the buttermilk. The yogurt can be unfermented or sour (fermented), depending on your taste.

Note: As the buttermilk stew already contains buttermilk, some people skip buttermilk with this lunch. However, if you feel like it, go ahead and have it.

QUINOA LUNCH

Cooked Quinoa • Green Sorrel (Khatta Palak) Dal • Ridge Gourd Curry • Coconut-Curd Chutney • Tomato Rasam • Buttermilk (optional)

COOKED QUINOA

Quinoa has less carbohydrates and a lower glycemic index. It is gluten free and rich in fiber, minerals, vitamins, antioxidants and nutrients, making it a diabetes-friendly food.

Ingredients
Quinoa:6 oz. (160 ml)

Directions
Cook the quinoa with 12 oz. (320 ml) of water until tender.

GREEN SORREL (KHATTA PALAK) DAL

Ingredients
Green Gram (moong dal): 3 oz. (80 ml)

Sorrel leaves: 1 bunch

Green chilis: 2, split

Tempering ingredients
Mustard seeds: 1/8 teaspoon

Cumin seeds: 1/8 teaspoon

Black gram: 1/8 teaspoon

Dry red chili: 1

Turmeric: a pinch

Curry leaves: 2 stalks

Asafetida: a pinch

Garlic: 2 cloves (optional)

Oil: 2 tablespoons

Salt: sufficient quantity

Directions
Cook the green gram, green sorrel leaves, and split green chilis in a sufficient quantity of water. Add salt in the final stages of cooking.

Temper the dal with the tempering ingredients after roasting them in oil.

RIDGE GOURD CURRY

Ingredients
Ridge gourd: 400 grams (about 1 lb.)

Onions: 2

Dry red chilis: 2

Oil: 2 tablespoons

Salt: sufficient quantity

Directions
Peel the ridge gourds and cut them into pieces.

Grind onions along with dry red chilis and salt into a paste.

Pour oil in a saucepan and cook the ridge gourd, adding the onion-red chili paste. Cook with the lid closed for 20 minutes. Occasionally stir the curry.

COCONUT-CURD CHUTNEY

Ingredients

Grated coconut: 12 oz. (320 ml)

Semi-thick curd: 12 oz. (320 ml)

Salt: sufficient

Tempering ingredients

Mustard seeds: 1/8 teaspoon

Dry red chilis: 2

Curry leaves: 2 stalks

Oil: 2 teaspoons

Asafetida: a pinch

Directions

Mix the grated coconut with semi-thick curd (yogurt). Add salt to taste.

Temper it with the tempering ingredients after frying them in oil.

TOMATO RASAM

Ingredients

Very small tomatoes: 4

Coriander leaves: a small quantity

Salt: sufficient quantity

Pepper powder: ¼ teaspoon

Turmeric powder: a pinch

Lemon juice: 1 tablespoon

Tempering ingredients

Mustard seeds: 1/8 teaspoon

Red chilis: 1

Cumin: 1/8 teaspoon

Asafetida: a pinch

Curry leaves: 2 stalks

Oil: 2 teaspoons

Directions

Boil the tomatoes in 18 oz. (480 ml) of water, adding salt, pepper powder, turmeric powder, and coriander leaves. When the rasam has fully boiled, add lemon juice.

Temper the rasam with the tempering ingredients after frying them in oil.

BUTTERMILK MADE FROM YOGURT (OPTIONAL)

Ingredients

Curd (Yogurt): 6 oz (160ml)

Salt: sufficient quantity (optional)

Directions

Mix 12 oz. (320 ml) of water in curd (yogurt) to prepare the buttermilk. The yogurt can be unfermented or sour (fermented), depending on your taste.

FOXTAIL MILLET LUNCH

Cooked Foxtail Millet • Fenugreek Leaf Dal • Tindora Curry with Onion Paste • Yellow Cucumber Chutney • Mixed Vegetable Stew • Buttermilk (optional)

COOKED FOXTAIL MILLET

Foxtail millet has a low glycemic index with a low carbohydrate content. It is enriched with many nutrients, minerals and vitamins. A lunch with foxtail millet along with vegetables and dal is thus tasty and beneficial for Type 2 diabetics.

Ingredients
Foxtail Millet: 6 oz. (160 ml)

Directions
Wash the foxtail millet and soak it in 15 oz. (400 ml) of water for 12 hours. Cook the soaked millet in the same water in a pressure cooker and keep it aside as you prepare the other dishes.

. . . .

FENUGREEK (METHI) LEAF DAL

Ingredients
Pigeon pea (toor dal): 3 oz. (80 ml)
Fenugreek leaves: one bunch, chopped
Salt: sufficient quantity

Tempering ingredients
Oil: 1 tablespoon
Mustard seeds: 1/8 teaspoon
Black gram: 1/3 teaspoon
Dry red chilis: 2
Curry leaves: 2 stalks
Asafetida: 1 pinch
Turmeric powder: 1 pinch

Directions
Wash and chop the fenugreek leaves. Cook the toor dal with the fenugreek in sufficient water. Add salt to taste.

Temper the dal with the tempering ingredients after roasting them in oil.

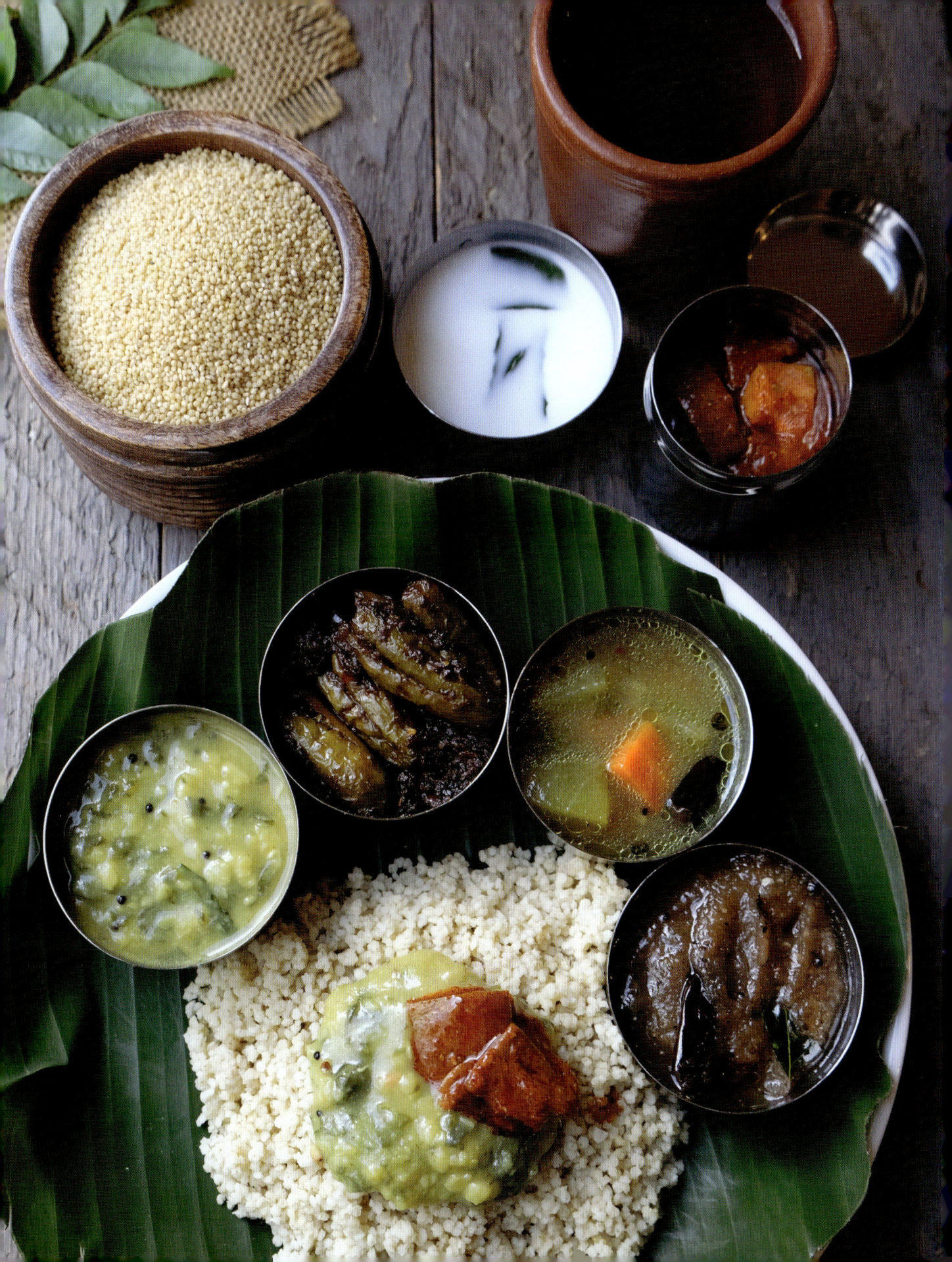

TINDORA CURRY WITH ONION PASTE

Ingredients

Tindora (ivy gourd): ¼ kg (about ½ pound)

Onions: 2

Dry red chilis: 3

Salt: sufficient quantity

Oil: 4 tablespoons

Directions

Wash the tindora thoroughly. Slit them on 4 sides.

Grind the onions and dry red chilis together into a paste. Add salt to taste.

Stuff the paste into the tindora and fry them in oil in a saucepan. Add water and let them cook for 5 minutes.

Put a lid on top of the saucepan and cook for another 20 minutes. Stir the curry with a spoon now and then. Add more water as needed for the curry to cook sufficiently.

YELLOW CUCUMBER CHUTNEY

Ingredients

Yellow cucumber: 1 medium sized

Tamarind: a small quantity

Dry red chilis: 3

Salt: sufficient quantity

Tempering ingredients

Mustard seeds: ⅛ teaspoon

Black gram: ⅓ teaspoon

Dry red chilis: 2, roasted

Curry leaves: 2 stalks

Asafetida: 1 pinch

Turmeric powder: 1 pinch

Oil: 1 tablespoon

Directions

Pierce the yellow cucumber once with a knife and roast it over a flame.

After it cools down, peel it and mash the pulp in a bowl. Taste it to make sure it's not bitter as some yellow cucumbers can be bitter.

Grind the pulp with tamarind, roasted dry red chilies, and salt. Temper the mixture with the tempering ingredients after roasting them in oil. Serve and enjoy.

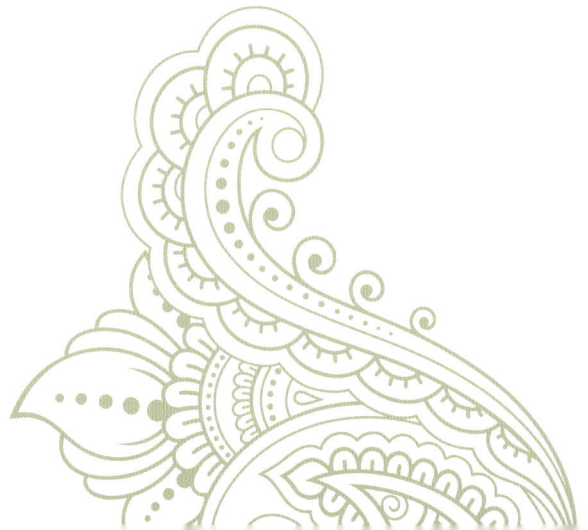

MIXED VEGETABLE STEW

Even if some of the vegetables are not available, you can make this stew, and the taste will not be affected.

Ingredients

Bottle gourd: ¼ piece

Radish: 1 (optional)

Carrot: 1

Onion: 1

Fenugreek seeds: ¼ teaspoon

Coriander leaves: a small amount, chopped

Turmeric powder: a small quantity

Green chilis: 1, split into halves

Salt: sufficient quantity

Jaggery: a small quantity

Tamarind juice: sufficient quantity

Chickpea powder: 1 teaspoon

Tempering Ingredients

Mustard seeds: $1/8$ teaspoon

Dry red chilis: 2, cut into pieces

Asafetida: 1 pinch

Curry leaves: 2 stalks

Oil: 1 tablespoon

Directions

Cut the bottle gourd, radish, carrot, and onion into pieces and boil them in 30 oz. (800 ml) of water. When they are boiling, add the fenugreek seeds, chopped coriander leaves, turmeric powder, green chili split into halves, salt, jaggery and tamarind juice.

After the stew has boiled fully, temper it with the tempering ingredients after roasting them in oil.

Add the chickpea powder after the stew cools down to adjust its taste and consistency.

BUTTERMILK MADE FROM YOGURT (OPTIONAL)

Ingredients

Curd (Yogurt): 6 oz (160ml)

Salt: sufficient quantity (optional)

Directions

Mix 12 oz. (320 ml) of water in curd (yogurt) to prepare the buttermilk. The yogurt can be unfermented or sour (fermented), depending on your taste.

SORGHUM (JOWAR) LUNCH

Cooked Jowar • Spinach Dal • Bottle Gourd Curry • Brinjal Curd Chutney • Pigeon Pea Stew • Buttermilk (optional)

COOKED SORGHUM (JOWAR)

Jowar has a low glycemic index and is rich in vitamins, minerals, nutrients and fiber, making it a recommended food for people with diabetes.

Ingredients

Jowar (sorghum): 6 oz. (160 ml)

Directions

Wash the jowar (sorghum) thoroughly and soak in 30 oz. (800 ml) of water for 12 hours. Drain the water from the jowar, then grind it a little to remove the outer rind. Do not grind it into flour.

Cook the ground jowar in 30 oz. (800 ml) of water adding salt. Using a pressure cooker is advisable.

· ·

SPINACH DAL

Ingredients

Pigeon pea (toor dal): 3 oz. (80 ml)

Spinach: 1 bunch, cut into pieces

Green chilis: 2, cut into pieces

Garlic: 4 cloves (optional)

Tamarind: Sufficient quantity

Turmeric powder: a pinch

Salt: sufficient quantity

Tempering ingredients

Mustard seeds: ⅛ teaspoon

Cumin seeds: ⅛ teaspoon

Dry red chilis: 2, cut into pieces

Black gram: ½ teaspoon

Asafetida: a pinch

Curry leaves: 2 stalks

Oil: 1 tablespoon

Directions

Wash the pigeon pea and spinach, cut into pieces.

Cook the pigeon pea and spinach in 18 oz. (480 ml) of water along with the green chilis, garlic cloves (optional), tamarind, and turmeric powder. Add salt after the dal has fully cooked. Depending on your taste, you can add more water.

Temper the dal with the tempering ingredients after frying them in oil. Your delicious spinach dal is ready.

BOTTLE GOURD CURRY

Ingredients

Bottle gourd: 1 medium-sized
Tamarind juice: 1.5 oz. (40 ml)
Salt: sufficient quantity

Tempering ingredients

Mustard seeds: $1/8$ teaspoon
Cumin seeds: $1/8$ teaspoon
Chickpea dal: $1/3$ teaspoon
Black gram: $1/3$ teaspoon
Dry red chilis: 2, cut into pieces
Green chilis: 1, cut into pieces
Asafetida: a pinch
Curry leaves: 2 stalks
Oil: 1 tablespoon

Directions

Peel the bottle gourd, cut it into small pieces, and cook them fully in a little water.

Roast the tempering ingredients, except for the green chili, in oil. Add the green chili cut into pieces to the roasted ingredients and continue roasting for a few minutes.

Add the cooked bottle gourd, tamarind juice, and salt to the roasted tempering ingredients, and keep the curry on a low flame for two minutes.

. . . .

BRINJAL CURD CHUTNEY

Ingredients

Brinjal (eggplant): 1 large, black or white
Curd (yogurt): 12 oz. (320 ml)
Green chilis: 2, cut into pieces
Salt: sufficient quantity

Tempering ingredients

Mustard seeds: $1/8$ teaspoon
Asafetida: a pinch
Dry red chilis: 2, cut into pieces
Curry leaves: 2 stalks
Oil: 1 tablespoon
Coriander leaves: a small amount

Directions

Pierce the brinjal with a knife and roast it over a flame. Then peel it and extract the pulp.

In a bowl, add the brinjal pulp to the curd, sour or unfermented, as per your taste. Mix the two into a smooth chutney using your hand. Add the green chilis and salt.

Temper the chutney with the tempering ingredients after roasting them in oil.

Garnish the chutney with coriander leaves, then serve and enjoy.

PIGEON PEA (TOOR DAL) STEW

Ingredients

Pigeon pea (toor dal): 3 oz. (80 ml)

Tamarind juice: 3 oz. (80 ml)

Jaggery: a small piece

Green chili: 1, split

Salt: sufficient quantity

Turmeric: a pinch

Tempering ingredients

Mustard seeds: 1/8 teaspoon

Dry red chilis: 2

Cumin seeds: 1/8 teaspoon

Curry leaves: 2 stalks

Asafetida: a pinch

Garlic: 4 cloves (optional)

Oil: 1 tablespoon

Directions

Wash the pigeon pea and cook it in sufficient volume of water. After it is softly cooked, add the tamarind juice, jaggery, turmeric, split green chili, and salt, and cook for 5 minutes. Add water if needed.

Temper the mixture with the tempering ingredients after roasting them in oil.

. . . .

BUTTERMILK MADE FROM YOGURT (OPTIONAL)

Ingredients

Curd (Yogurt): 6 oz (160ml)

Salt: sufficient quantity (optional)

Directions

Mix 12 oz. (320 ml) of water in curd (yogurt) to prepare the buttermilk. The yogurt can be unfermented or sour (fermented), depending on your taste.

CAULIFLOWER RICE LUNCH

Cooked Cauliflower Rice • Yellow Cucumber Dal • Taro Root Curry • Ridge Gourd Peel Chutney • Green Gram (moong dal) Stew • Buttermilk (optional)

COOKED CAULIFLOWER RICE

Cauliflower is rich in folate, vitamins B, C, K, and fiber. It contains many nutrients, minerals and antioxidants. Above all, it has a very low carbohydrate content and a low glycemic index, making it the best choice for Type 2 diabetics.

Ingredients

Cauliflower rice: 12 oz. (320 ml)

Directions

Divide a large cauliflower into florets. Wash them thoroughly in warm water for 2 minutes, then allow them to dry for a few hours on a sheet of paper. Grate the florets to produce cauliflower rice.

Cook the cauliflower rice in a saucepan on a medium flame, sprinkling only a tablespoon of water on it.

YELLOW CUCUMBER DAL

Ingredients

Pigeon Pea (toor dal): 3 oz. (80 ml)
Yellow cucumber: 1
Green chilis: 1, split
Coriander leaves: a small amount
Salt: sufficient quantity
Lemon juice: 2 tablespoons

Tempering ingredients

Mustard seeds: $1/8$ teaspoon
Black gram: $1/3$ teaspoon
Dry red chilis: 2, cut into pieces
Asafetida: a pinch
Turmeric: a pinch
Oil: 1 Tablespoon

Directions

Wash the pigeon pea. Peel a yellow cucumber and cut it into pieces.

Place both the pigeon pea and yellow cucumber pieces in a pressure cooker. Add the split green chili and coriander leaves. Cook the ingredients in a sufficient volume of water to ensure that the dal is thin. After it is fully cooked, add salt and lemon juice.

Temper the dal with the tempering ingredients after roasting them in oil. Garnish the dal with coriander leaves.

TARO ROOT CURRY

Ingredients

Taro roots: 250 grams (about ½ lb.)

Mustard seeds: ⅛ teaspoon

Cumin seeds: ⅛ teaspoon

Black gram: ½ teaspoon

Curry leaves: 2 stalks

Dry red chilis: 3, cut into pieces

Asafetida: a pinch

Salt: sufficient quantity

Oil: 4 tablespoons

Directions

Cut the taro roots and boil them until they are completely cooked. Peel the boiled roots and cut them into medium-sized pieces.

In a frying pan, fry the mustard seeds, black gram, cumin seeds, dry red chilis cut into pieces, curry leaves, and asafetida in oil. Add the cut taro root pieces and salt to taste. Cook on a medium flame with the lid closed. (Note: As the taro root has already been boiled, it takes only three minutes to completely cook the dish.)

RIDGE GOURD PEEL CHUTNEY

Ingredients

Ridge gourds: 3

Oil: 2 tablespoons

Tamarind juice: 3 oz. (80 ml)

Jaggery: a small piece (optional)

Green chilis: 2

Dry red chilis: 3

Salt: sufficient quantity

Tempering ingredients

Mustard seeds: ⅛ teaspoon

Cumin seeds: ⅛ teaspoon

Dry red chilis: 1, cut into pieces

Garlic: 2 cloves (optional)

Black gram: ⅓ teaspoon

Turmeric: a pinch

Asafetida: a pinch

Oil: 1 tablespoon

Directions

Peel the ridge gourds. Heat the oil in a frying pan and fry the gourd peel. Don't use the ridge gourd pulp, as the peel itself, without the pulp, makes a tasty chutney. You can use the pulp later for making a curry.

Grind the fried and cooled ridge gourd peel along with tamarind, jaggery (optional), salt, green chilis and dry red chilis into a paste.

Temper the chutney with the tempering ingredients after frying them in oil. Your yummy ridge gourd peel chutney is ready to be served and enjoyed.

GREEN GRAM (MOONG DAL) STEW

Ingredients

Green gram: 3 oz. (80 ml)

Tamarind juice: 3 oz. (80 ml)

Jaggery: a small piece

Green chili: 1, split

Turmeric powder: a little

Salt: sufficient quantity

Tempering ingredients

Mustard seeds: $\frac{1}{8}$ teaspoon

Dry red chilis: 2

Asafetida: a pinch

Garlic: 4 cloves (optional)

Curry leaves: 2 stalks

Oil: 1 tablespoon

Directions

Wash the green gram and cook it in sufficient volume of water.

Add the split green chili, tamarind juice, jaggery, turmeric, and salt and cook for 5 minutes. Add water if necessary.

After the stew is fully cooked, temper it with the tempering ingredients after roasting them in oil.

BUTTERMILK MADE FROM YOGURT (OPTIONAL)

Ingredients

Curd (Yogurt): 6 oz (160ml)

Salt: sufficient quantity (optional)

Directions

Mix 12 oz. (320 ml) of water in curd (yogurt) to prepare the buttermilk. The yogurt can be unfermented or sour (fermented), depending on your taste.

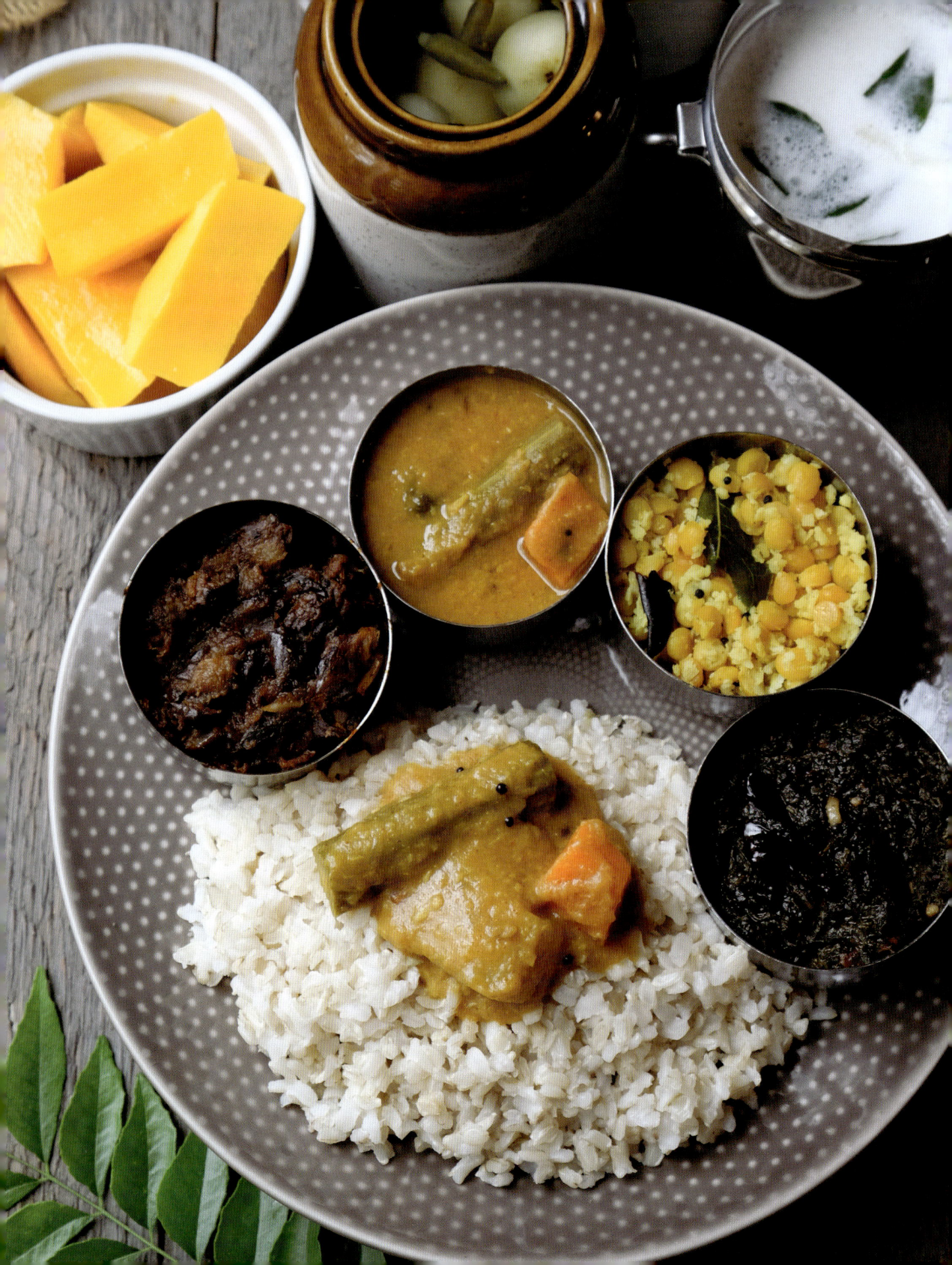

BROWN RICE LUNCH

Cooked Brown Rice • Coconut Chickpea (Chana Dal) • Brinjal Onion Fry • Sorrel Leaf Chutney • Sambar • Buttermilk (optional)

COOKED BROWN RICE

Brown rice has less carbohydrate content and lower glycemic index, making it a diabetes friendly food.

Ingredients
Brown rice: 6 oz. (160 ml)

Directions
Soak the brown rice for about 8 hours and cook it in a pressure cooker.

- -

COCONUT CHICKPEA (CHANA DAL)

Ingredients
Chickpea dal: 6 oz. (160 ml)
Grated coconut: 12 oz. (320 ml)
Salt: sufficient quantity

Tempering ingredients
Mustard seeds: 1/8 teaspoon
Black gram: 1/3 teaspoon
Chickpea dal: 1/3 teaspoon
Asafetida: 1 pinch
Dry red chilis: 1
Curry leaves: 2 stalks
Oil: 1 tablespoon

Directions
Cook the chickpea dal in a sufficient quantity of water until all the water evaporates. Add salt as needed.

Roast the tempering ingredients in oil. Add the roasted items to the boiled chickpea dal.

Add the grated coconut into the chickpea dal and fry it for 3 minutes on a low flame. This delicious dish is now ready to serve.

- -

BRINJAL ONION FRY

Ingredients
Brinjals (eggplants): 250 grams (about ½ lb.)
Onions: 2, cut into pieces
Oil: 3 tablespoons
Dry red chili cumin powder: ½ teaspoon
Salt: sufficient quantity

Directions
Wash the brinjals and cut them into pieces. Heat the oil in a frying pan. Add the cut brinjals and fry them on a medium flame, closing the pan with a lid. Once the brinjal is roasted by 75%, add the onions cut into pieces and fry the mixture for another 5 minutes in the closed pan to reduce the amount of oil needed.

Once the curry is fully cooked and roasted, add the dry red chili cumin powder and salt to taste.

SORREL LEAF CHUTNEY

Ingredients

Sorrel leaves: 1 bunch

Dry red chilis: 5

Green chilis: 5

Tamarind: Sufficient quantity

Salt: sufficient quantity

Oil: 3 tablespoons

Tempering ingredients

Mustard seeds: 1/8 teaspoon

Black gram: 1/3 teaspoon

Garlic: 4 cloves (optional)

Oil: 1 tablespoon

Curry leaves: 2 stalks

Dry red chilis: 1, cut into pieces

Asafetida: 1 pinch

Directions

Wash the sorrel leaves and allow them to dry completely. Then fry the sorrel leaves along with the dry red chilis in oil.

Grind the above ingredients with the green chilis, tamarind, and salt. Depending on the sourness of the sorrel leaves, you can adjust the quantity of tamarind and the number of green and dry red chilis to your taste.

Temper the chutney with the tempering ingredients after roasting them in oil. Add garlic (optional) in the final stages of roasting.

SAMBAR

See recipe for Sambar on page 30.

BUTTERMILK MADE FROM YOGURT (OPTIONAL)

Ingredients

Curd (Yogurt): 6 oz (160ml)

Salt: sufficient quantity (optional)

Directions

Mix 12 oz. (320 ml) of water in curd (yogurt) to prepare the buttermilk. The yogurt can be unfermented or sour (fermented), depending on your taste.

BARNYARD MILLET LUNCH

Cooked Barnyard Millet • Pigeon Pea (toor dal) • Brinjal-Ginger Curry • Tomato Chutney • Amaranth Stew • Buttermilk (optional)

COOKED BARNYARD MILLET

Barnyard millet has a glycemic index between 42 and 50, which is considered low, so it doesn't raise blood sugar levels. It has a high amount of protein, healthy fats, and fiber plus many minerals, nutrients, and vitamins, making it a good choice for people with Type 2 diabetes.

Ingredients

Barnyard millet: 6 oz. (160 ml)

Directions

Wash the barnyard millet thoroughly, then soak it for 12 hours.

Drain the water completely. Add 12 oz. (320 ml) of fresh water and cook the millet on a high flame, closing the saucepan with a lid.

Stir the millets two or three times during the cooking process. Lower the flame in the final stages of cooking and you will have a nicely cooked barnyard millet.

PIGEON PEA (TOOR DAL)

Ingredients

Pigeon pea (toor dal): 3 oz. (80 ml)

Ghee: 1 teaspoon

Salt: sufficient quantity

Directions

Wash the toor dal, then roast it briefly in ghee and finally cook it in water. After it is fully cooked, add salt.

BRINJAL-GINGER CURRY

Ingredients

Brinjal: 250 grams (about ½ lb.)

Gringer: a small piece

Green chilis: 2

Mustard seeds: ⅓ teaspoon

Black gram: ½ teaspoon

Chickpea dal: ½ teaspoon

Dry red chilis: 1, cut into pieces

Asafetida: a pinch

Turmeric: a pinch

Curry leaves: 2 stalks

Oil: 1 tablespoon

Tamarind juice: 2 oz. (50 ml)

Chickpea flour: ½ teaspoon

Salt: sufficient quantity

Directions

Cut the brinjals, preferably white, into pieces. Boil the pieces in a sufficient quantity of water. Make sure the water completely evaporates and only the boiled brinjal remains in the saucepan.

Grind ginger and green chilies into a paste.

Roast the mustard seeds, black gram, dry red chilis, chickpea dal, asafetida, curry leaves and turmeric in oil.

Add the ginger-chili paste, tamarind juice and salt along with cooked brinjal to the above roasted ingredients, and keep it on a low flame for 3 minutes.

Add the chickpea flour to the curry to bring about a good taste and consistency.

TINDORA CHUTNEY

Ingredients

Oil: 3 tablespoons

Fenugreek seeds: 1 teaspoon

Mustard seeds: 1 teaspoon

Black gram: 1 teaspoon

Chickpea dal: 1 teaspoon

Tindora: 200 grams (about ½ lb.), cut into pieces

Green chilis: 10

Tamarind: a small piece

Salt: sufficient quantity

Tempering ingredients

Mustard seeds: ⅛ teaspoon

Cumin seeds: ⅛ teaspoon

Curry leaves: 2 stalks • Asafetida: a pinch

Black gram: ⅓ teaspoon • Oil: 1 tablespoon

Turmeric: a pinch

Directions

Heat one tablespoon of oil in a saucepan and lightly roast half a teaspoon of fenugreek seeds. After they are roasted to a half extent, add half a teaspoon of mustard seeds, black gram, and chickpea dal and roast them all. Remove the ingredients and allow them to cool. Then grind them into a fine powder and set aside.

Heat two tablespoons of oil in a saucepan and add the tindora cut into pieces with the green chilis, and fry them, covering the saucepan with a lid. Keep them on a low flame for a few minutes so that they will cook fully.

Add the tamarind and keep the mixture in the saucepan for one more minute. After all the ingredients cool down, combine them with the previously ground powder and salt, and grind it all to a coarse paste.

Temper the chutney with the tempering ingredients after roasting them in oil.

Serve and enjoy this distinctive chutney.

AMARANTH STEW

Ingredients

Amaranth leaves: 1 bunch

Tamarind juice: 6 oz. (160 ml)

Brinjals: 1, cut into pieces

Onions: 1, cut into pieces

Green chilis: 1, split

Coriander leaves: small amount, chopped

Turmeric powder: a pinch

Jaggery: 1 small piece

Salt: sufficient quantity

Rice flour: 1 teaspoon

Mustard powder: ½ teaspoon

Tempering ingredients

Oil: 1 tablespoon

Mustard seeds: $1/8$ teaspoon

Cumin seeds: $1/8$ teaspoon

Dry red chilis: 2, cut into pieces

Asafetida: a pinch

Directions

Wash the amaranth and cut it into pieces. Boil these in water, adding tamarind juice, brinjal cut into pieces, onion cut into pieces, split green chili, coriander leaves, turmeric powder, jaggery, and salt.

Once the mixture is fully cooked, temper the stew with the tempering ingredients after they have been fried in oil.

Mix the rice flour in a small amount of water, avoiding lumps, and add it to the stew. Stir thoroughly.

After the stew has cooled down, add the mustard powder and mix well.

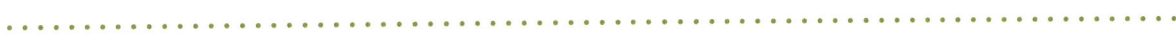

BUTTERMILK MADE FROM YOGURT (OPTIONAL)

Ingredients

Curd (Yogurt): 6 oz (160ml)

Salt: sufficient quantity (optional)

Directions

Mix 12 oz. (320 ml) of water in curd (yogurt) to prepare the buttermilk. The yogurt can be unfermented or sour (fermented), depending on your taste.

ALMOND POORI LUNCH
Almond Poori • Bombay Chutney • Buttermilk (optional)

ALMOND POORI

As pooris are associated with oil, it is advisable to eat them in moderation with more curry. If you are a little unsatisfied with the quantity of this lunch, you can eat a sufficient amount of salad with a spicy dressing to make your diet complete.

Almond flour is rich in protein, nutrients, fiber, antioxidants and healthy fats. It has less carbohydrates, and thus a low glycemic index. It is also gluten free. This makes it highly recommended food for people with Type 2 diabetes.

Ingredients
Almond flour: 7 oz. (200 ml)

Xanthan gum: 1 teaspoon

Oil: 8 oz. (250 ml)

Ghee: 1 tablespoon

Salt: sufficient quantity

Directions
Mix the almond flour with xanthan gum and salt in a bowl. Make it into a dough, adding a tablespoon of ghee and 1½ teaspoons of water.

Keep the dough in a bowl for 15 minutes, then knead it vigorously using both hands. Divide the dough into small balls.

Place each ball on a transparent plastic sheet and cover it with another sheet. Then make the balls into puris using a rolling pin to flatten the dough.

Heat oil in a frying pan and keep it on medium flame. Once the oil is fully hot, fry the puris softly or crisply per your preference.

The suggested curry is Bombay chutney.

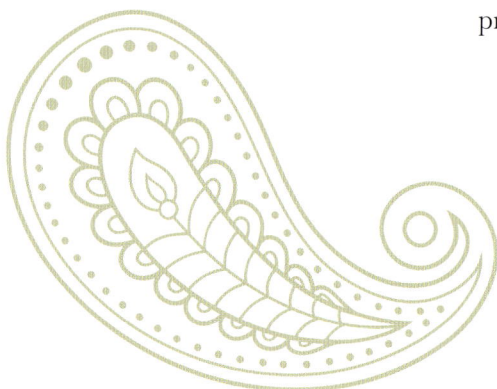

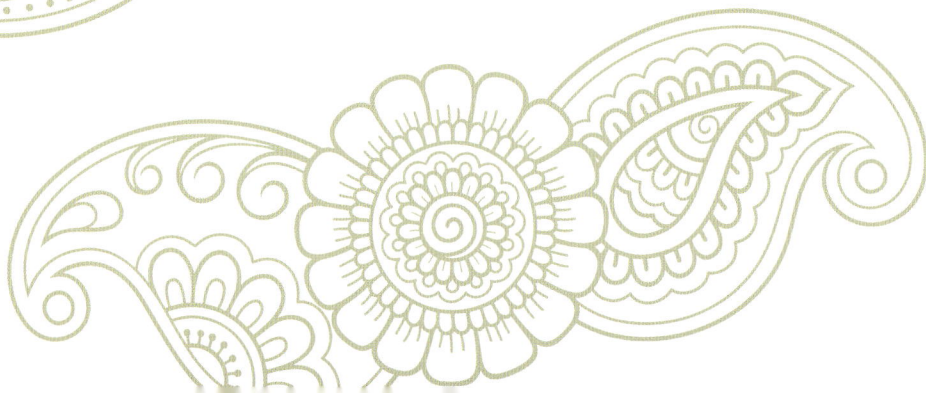

BOMBAY CHUTNEY

Though it is called a chutney, this recipe is actually a curry. The consistency of the dish can vary according to your taste.

Ingredients

Chickpea flour: 2 to 3 tablespoons

Onions: 3, cut into slices

Tomatoes: 2, cut into pieces

Green chilis: 3, cut into pieces

Ginger: a medium sized piece

Black gram: ½ teaspoon

Chickpea dal: ½ teaspoon

Mustard seeds: ¼ teaspoon

Dry red chilis: 2

Garlic: 6 cloves, chopped (optional)

Curry leaves: 2 stalks

Asafetida: a pinch

Turmeric powder: a pinch

Oil: 2 tablespoons

Tamarind juice: 1.5 oz. (40 ml)

Salt: sufficient quantity

Coriander leaves: small amount

Directions

Cut the onions into long, thin slices. Cut the tomatoes, green chilis, and ginger into pieces. Set aside.

In a saucepan, fry the black gram, chickpea dal, mustard seeds, dry red chili, garlic cloves (optional), curry leaves, asafetida, and turmeric powder in oil.

Add the cut slices of onion and roast them a little. Add the ginger cut into small pieces, green chilies cut into pieces, and tomato cut into pieces and fry them together, adding salt, until they are sufficiently cooked.

Mix the chickpea flour thoroughly in 6 oz. (160 ml) water and add it to the above cooked ingredients.

Garnish the dish with coriander leaves.

BUTTERMILK MADE FROM YOGURT (OPTIONAL)

Ingredients

Curd (Yogurt): 6 oz (160ml)

Salt: sufficient quantity (optional)

Directions

Mix 12 oz. (320 ml) of water in curd (yogurt) to prepare the buttermilk. The yogurt can be unfermented or sour (fermented), depending on your taste.

For people who, under constraints of time, cannot prepare a meal with many dishes or a dish that takes a lot of time to make, I am providing what I call a Superfast Lunch. This recipe is a template that can be varied in many ways by choosing one of each ingredient to quickly make a one-dish nutritious lunch. The resulting meal will consist of fewer carbohydrates, making it highly recommended for people with Type 2 diabetes. Moreover, the taste is indescribable. You can also use this recipe for a dinner.

SUPERFAST LUNCH (BASIC RECIPE)

Ingredients

Choose one item from each category

Pearl millet/ little millet/ kodo millet/ quinoa/ brown rice: 6 oz. (160 ml)

Bottle gourd/ ridge gourd/ yellow cucumber/ okra/ tindora/ bitter gourd/ brinjal: 12 oz. (320 ml), chopped

Beans/ peas/ kidney beans: 6 oz. (160 ml)

Amaranth/spinach/ sorrel/ fenugreek: 12 oz. (320 ml), chopped

Radish/ carrot/ taro: 12 oz. (320 ml), chopped

Green gram (moong dal) / pigeon pea (toor dal): 3 oz. (80 ml)

Additional Ingredients

Green chilis: 2 teaspoons, cut into pieces

Lemon juice: 1 tablespoon

Salt: sufficient quantity

Directions

Cook one of the millets, quinoa, or brown rice. The cooking process for each of these is provided in the various lunch recipes. Next boil any one of the tubers, one of the beans options, one of the leafy vegetables, and one of the vegetables, all together in a sufficient volume of water. Add salt and green chilis.

Then cook either one of the dals in a sufficient volume of water, adding salt in the final stages of cooking.

Mix all the cooked ingredients together (cooked millet, cooked vegetables and dal), add lemon juice, and you will have a superfast meal.

Enjoy the meal with a lemon pickle, mango pickle, or any other pickle. The same meal can be taken for breakfast, lunch, or dinner.

Try different combinations of millets, beans, leafy vegetables, vegetables and lentils on different days for a change and prepare a different fast meal in the same way as the above meal.

You can have some buttermilk, as per your choice, at the end.

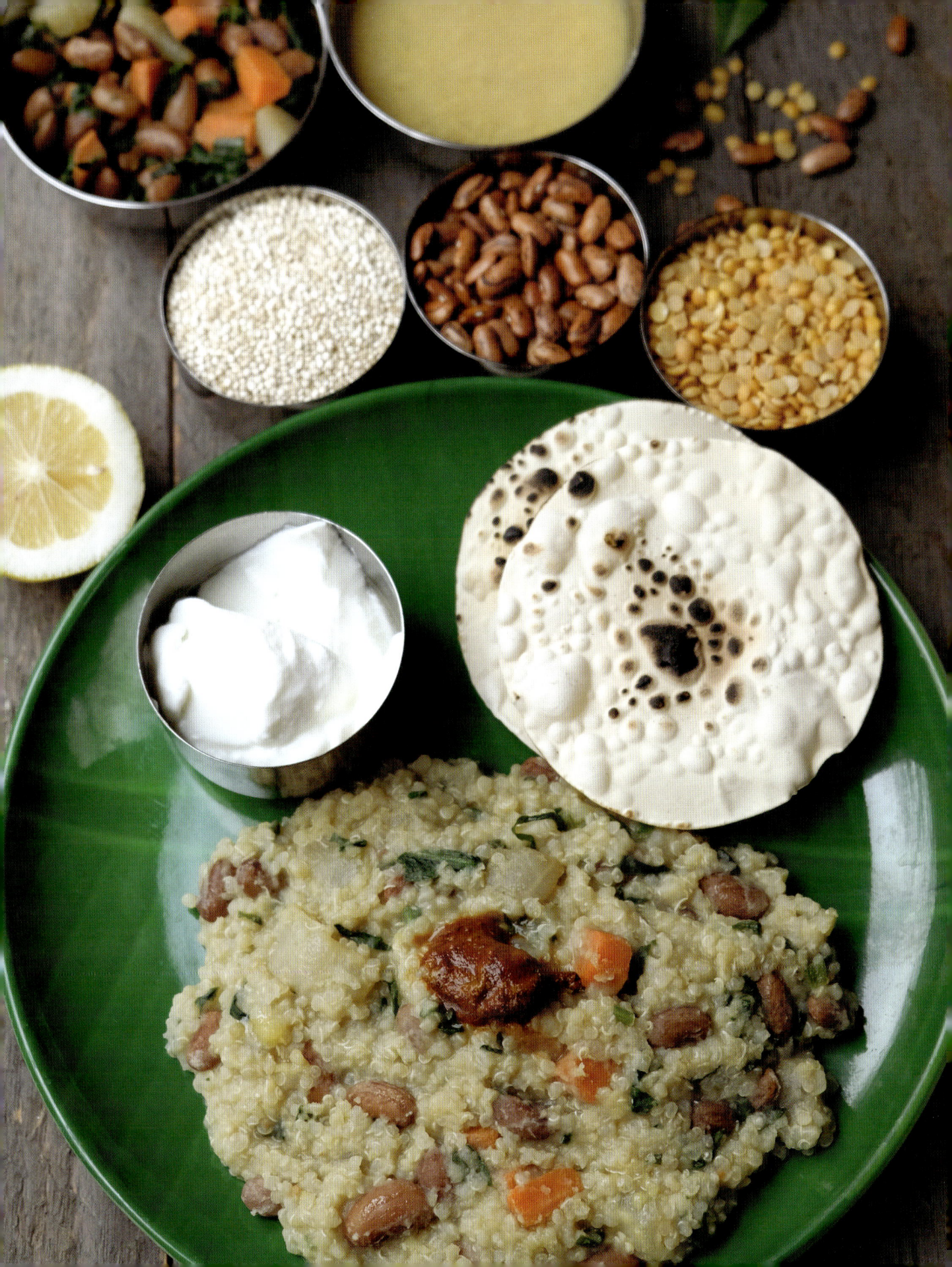

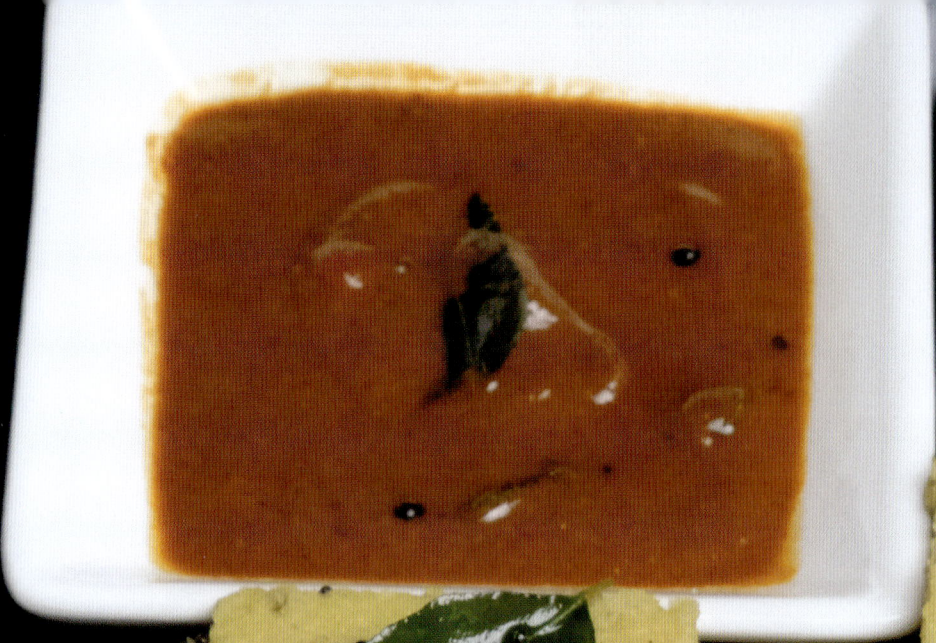

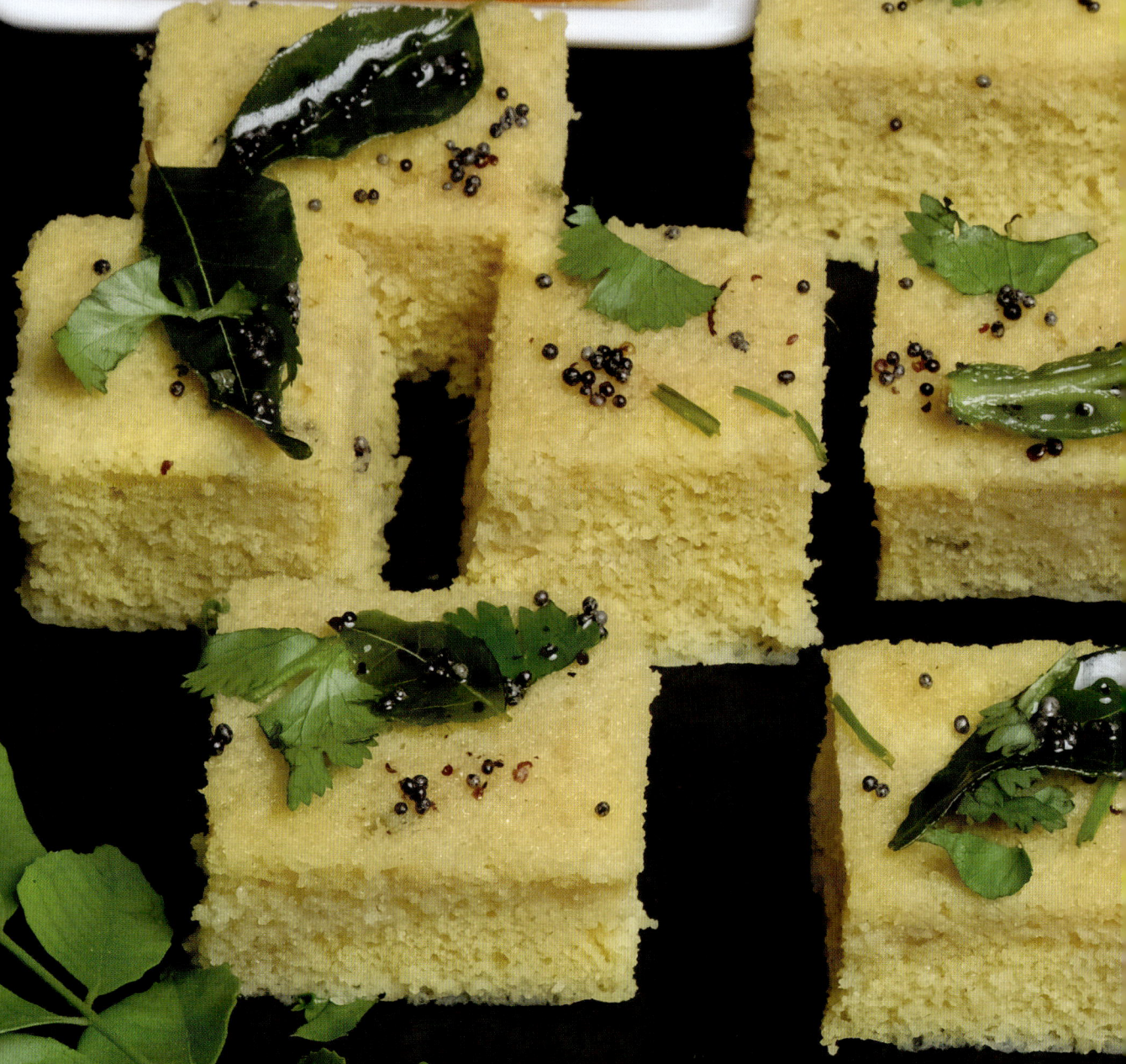

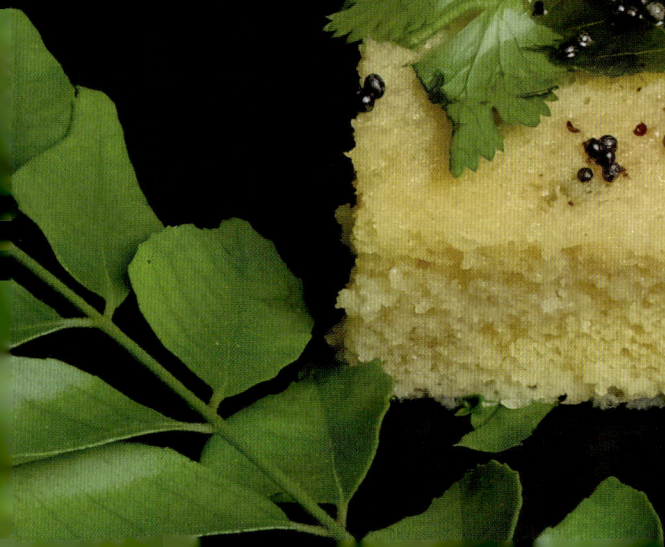

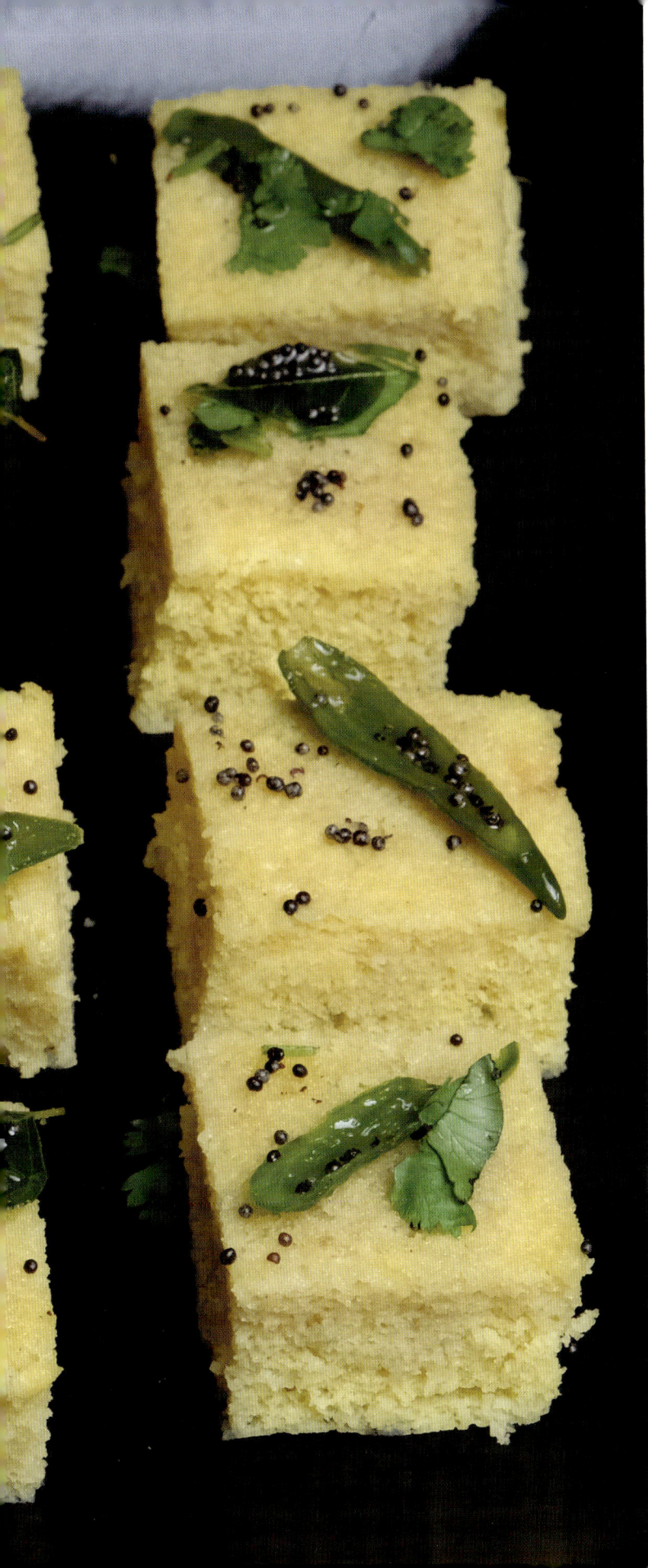

YUMMY DINNERS

Dhokla with Tamarind Chutney

BARLEY ROTI

Barley has a very low glycemic index (30). It has a good amount of fiber, so it slows down how fast the stomach empties, thus keeping cholesterol and blood sugar levels in control.

Ingredients

Barley flour: 12 oz. (320 ml)

Salt: sufficient quantity

Ghee: 1 tablespoon

Directions

Put the barley flour and salt in 6 oz. (160 ml) boiling water and let it stay for some time. Turn off the flame and let the mixture cool down.

Make the mixture into a dough and knead it vigorously using both hands.

Using a fistful of dough, make lemon-sized balls. Then using a chapati board and a roller pin, flatten the balls into rotis and fry them in ghee. No oil is needed.

The curry suggested is tomato onion.

. . . .

TOMATO ONION CURRY

Ingredients

Onions: 2, cut into pieces

Tomatoes: 4, cut into pieces

Green chilis: 2, cut into pieces

Oil: 2 tablespoons

Tamarind juice: 2 tablespoons

Salt: sufficient quantity

Dry red chili powder: ½ teaspoon

Coriander leaves: a small bunch

Tempering ingredients

Mustard seeds: $1/8$ teaspoon

Black gram: $1/3$ teaspoon

Red chilis: 1

Asafetida: ¼ teaspoon

Curry leaves: 2 stalks

Turmeric: ¼ teaspoon

Oil: 1 tablespoon

Directions

Lightly fry the onions, tomatoes, and green chilis in oil in a saucepan.

Add the tamarind juice and salt, and cook the vegetables for 3 additional minutes, closing the saucepan with a lid.

Add the coriander leaves and red chili powder. Keep the saucepan on the stove for another five minutes after turning off the fire to let the flavors mix.

Temper the mixture with the tempering ingredients after frying them in oil.

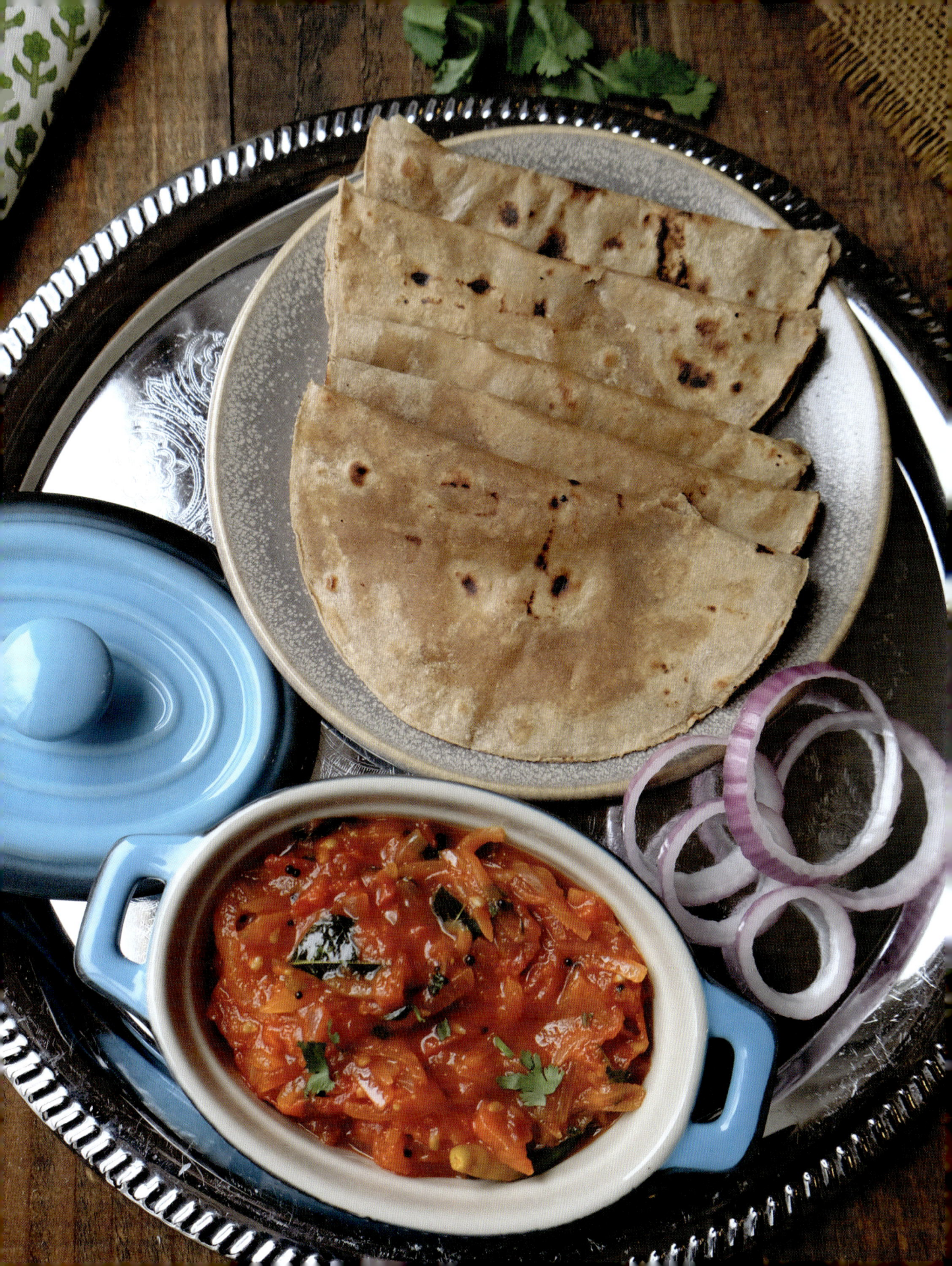

FOXTAIL MILLET DOSA

Ingredients

Foxtail Millet: 6 oz. (160 ml)

Black gram (urad dal): 3 oz. (80 ml)

Fenugreek seeds: 1 teaspoon

Flattened rice: 1.5 oz. (40 ml)

Salt: sufficient quantity

Oil: sufficient volume

Directions

Wash the foxtail millet thoroughly and soak it in water for 8 hours. Also wash black gram and soak it in water along with fenugreek for six hours. Also soak flattened rice for 10 minutes.

Grind the foxtail millet, black gram, flattened rice, and fenugreek together into a smooth dosa batter consistency, using a sufficient amount of water. Allow it to ferment for about 12 hours. Add salt to taste.

Heat a dosa pan on the stove. When it is fully hot, spread around a small amount of batter thinly on the pan. After one side is roasted, reverse it and roast it on the other side. You can use oil as needed.

Suggested chutney is white sesame.

WHITE SESAME CHUTNEY

Ingredients

White sesame seeds: 2 oz. (50 grams)

Dry red chilis: 4

Tamarind juice: 3 oz. (80 ml)

Salt: sufficient quantity

Jaggery: small piece

Tempering ingredients

Mustard seeds: 1/8 teaspoon

Cumin seeds: 1/8 teaspoon

Curry leaves: 2 stalks

Asafetida: a pinch

Oil: 1 tablespoon

Directions

Roast the sesame seeds along with the dry red chilis without using oil. Then grind the mixture, adding tamarind juice, a sufficient quantity of water, salt and jaggery. The chutney has to be a little thin.

Temper the chutney with the tempering ingredients after frying them in oil.

SORGHUM (JOWAR) ROTI

Sorghum has a low glycemic index and offers many other benefits for diabetics. Supplemented with the tasty black gram curry, it is not only a taste experience, but it also enhances the nutritional value of the food for Type 2 diabetics.

Ingredients
Sorghum (jowar) flour: 12 oz. (320 ml)
Salt: sufficient quantity

Directions
Mix the sorghum flour with 9 oz. (240 ml) of hot water, adding salt to taste. When it is semi-hot, make it into dough and knead it vigorously.

Use a fistful of dough to make lemon-sized balls. Put each ball on a wet cloth, and, using your hand, slowly press it into a thin roti.

Heat up a pan and place each roti with its cloth into the pan, then remove the cloth gently. Using a spatula, move the roti around the pan to roast it fully on both sides. No oil is needed for roasting the rotis. The curry suitable for jowar roti is a spicy black gram preparation.

BLACK GRAM, FENUGREEK (METHI) LEAF CURRY

Ingredients
Onions: 1, cut into pieces
Fenugreek leaves: 6 oz. (160 ml), chopped
Black gram husked: 6 oz. (160 ml)
Tomatoes: 2, cut into pieces
Coriander leaves: small amount, chopped
Salt: sufficient quantity

Tempering ingredients
Oil: 2 tablespoons
Mustard seeds: $1/8$ teaspoon
Cumin seeds: $1/8$ teaspoon
Asafetida: a pinch
Turmeric: a pinch
Green chilis: 5
Curry leaves: 2 stalks

Directions
In a saucepan, fry the tempering ingredients in oil. Then add the onion pieces and fenugreek leaves and roast them a little.

Add the black gram and roast it a little. Then add the tomatoes cut into pieces, 18 oz. (480 ml) of water, and cook the whole mixture for 20 minutes on a medium flame, covering the saucepan with a lid. Stir the curry now and then to ensure it cooks fully. Add salt and garnish with a small amount of chopped coriander leaves.

FINGER MILLET (RAGI) BURRITOS

Ingredients

Finger millet flour: 6 oz. (160 ml)

Wheat flour: 6 oz. (160 ml)

Oil: 1 tablespoon

Salt: sufficient quantity

Directions

Mix the finger millet flour and wheat flour in sufficient lukewarm water to make a sticky dough. Add salt. Knead the mixture vigorously with both hands.

From the mixture, make lemon-sized balls, then using a chapati board and rolling pin, flatten the balls into thin rotis that will become the wrapping for a burrito. Place each roti in a frying pan and roast it on both the sides without using oil. Stuff each one with the recipe below.

STUFFING FOR THE BURRITOS

Ingredients

Green gram sprouts: 6 oz. (160 ml)

Tomatoes: 2

Coriander: ½ bunch

Green chilis: 1

Onions: 2

Lemon juice: 2 tablespoons

Salt: sufficient quantity

Oil: 2 tablespoons

Directions

Heat the oil in a saucepan and add the green gram sprouts, tomatoes, onions, green chilis, and coriander leaves. Fry them for 5 minutes. Add salt and lemon juice. This will be the stuffing.

Place an amount of stuffing on each roti and roll it into round tubes like a burrito. Serve and enjoy.

No chutney is needed for this dish, though if you want, you can eat it with tomato ketchup.

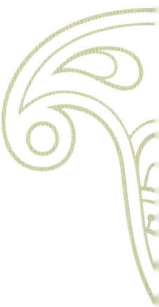

CURD QUINOA

Quinoa has many nutrients, fiber and iron, and is gluten free. Its glycemic index is low (53). It is a good choice for people with Type 2 diabetes. No chutney is needed for this recipe. However, if you want, you can eat it with a lime pickle or some other pickle.

Ingredients

Quinoa: 6 oz. (160 ml)
Curd: 18 oz. (480 ml)
Salt: sufficient quantity

Tempering ingredients

Oil: 1 tablespoon
Mustard seeds: 1/8 teaspoon
Black gram: 1/3 teaspoon
Chickpea dal: 1/3 teaspoon
Asafetida: a pinch
Fenugreek: 10 seeds only
Dry red chilis: 2, cut into pieces
Green chilis: 1, cut into pieces
Ginger: a small piece, grated
Curry leaves: 2 stalks
Coriander leaves: 2 tablespoons, chopped

Directions

Cook the quinoa in 12 oz. (240 ml) of water in a saucepan. When done, add the curd (yogurt) to the saucepan and salt to taste. Mix.

Heat oil in a frying pan and add the mustard seeds, black gram, chickpea dal, asafetida, fenugreek seeds, and dry red chilis cut into pieces. After they are roasted to some extent, add the green chilis cut into pieces, grated ginger, and curry leaves. Roast the mixture. After the tempering ingredients are fully roasted, add them to the quinoa curd.

Garnish the dish with coriander leaves, then serve and enjoy.

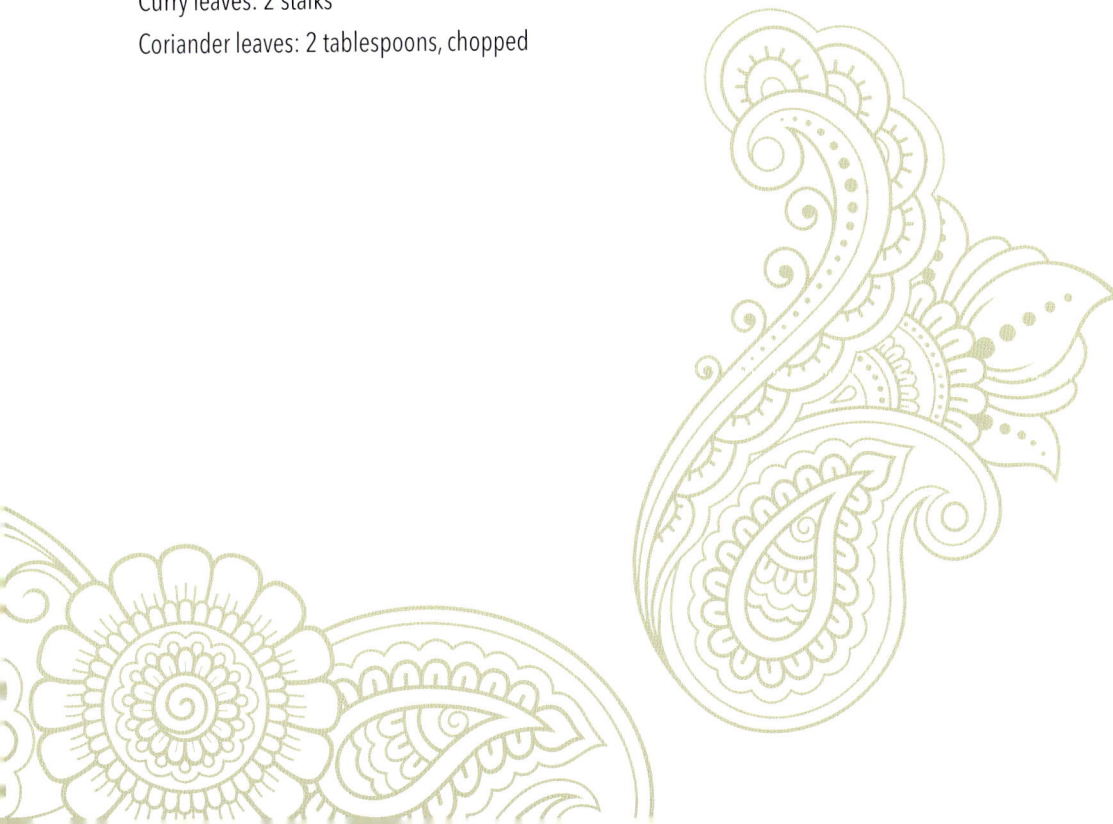

DHOKLA

Dhokla, being prepared with chickpea flour, has low glycemic index (44) and is rich in proteins, fiber, and vitamins besides being lower in calories and carbohydrates. This makes it a tasty and highly beneficial food for diabetics.

Ingredients

Green chilis: 2

Ginger: a small piece

Chickpea flour: 9 oz. (180 ml)

Salt: half a teaspoon

Sugar: half a teaspoon

Baking soda: ¼ teaspoon

Eno: ¾ teaspoon

Citric acid: 1 teaspoon

Turmeric powder: half a teaspoon

Oil: 1 tablespoon

Tempering ingredients

Mustard seeds: 1 teaspoon

Green chilis: 4

Curry leaves: 2 stalks

Salt: sufficient quantity

Sugar: 2 teaspoons

Directions

Grind the green chilis and ginger into a paste.

In a large bowl, mix well the chickpea flour, salt, sugar, baking soda, eno, citric acid, green chili-ginger paste, and turmeric powder.

Pour water slowly into the bowl and make a batter without lumps to idli consistency. Set the batter aside for 15 minutes.

Grease a saucepan all around on the inside to prevent the dhokla from sticking once it is cooked. Pour the entire batter in the saucepan and cook it using the steam method. This means that the saucepan should be put on a stand above a bigger saucepan containing boiling water. Cover the saucepan with a lid and steam the dhokla for 20 minutes. Let the dhokla remain in the saucepan for 10 more minutes.

Take the dhokla saucepan out of the larger saucepan below it and turn it upside down on a plate so that the entire dhokla comes out. Cut the dhokla into square-sized pieces about the size of Mysore bonda.

Heat oil in a frying pan and lightly roast the mustard seeds, then add the split green chilis and curry leaves and roast them further. Add a little water, half a teaspoon of salt, and 2 teaspoons of sugar to the roast and boil it to make a syrup. Once it is cooked, pour the syrup evenly on the dhoklas.

Note: The dhoklas can also be cooked in an idli cooker, but they will not be of their usual nice-looking square shape but roundish like idlis.

A tasty accompaniment for the dhoklas is tamarind chutney (recipe on page 80.)

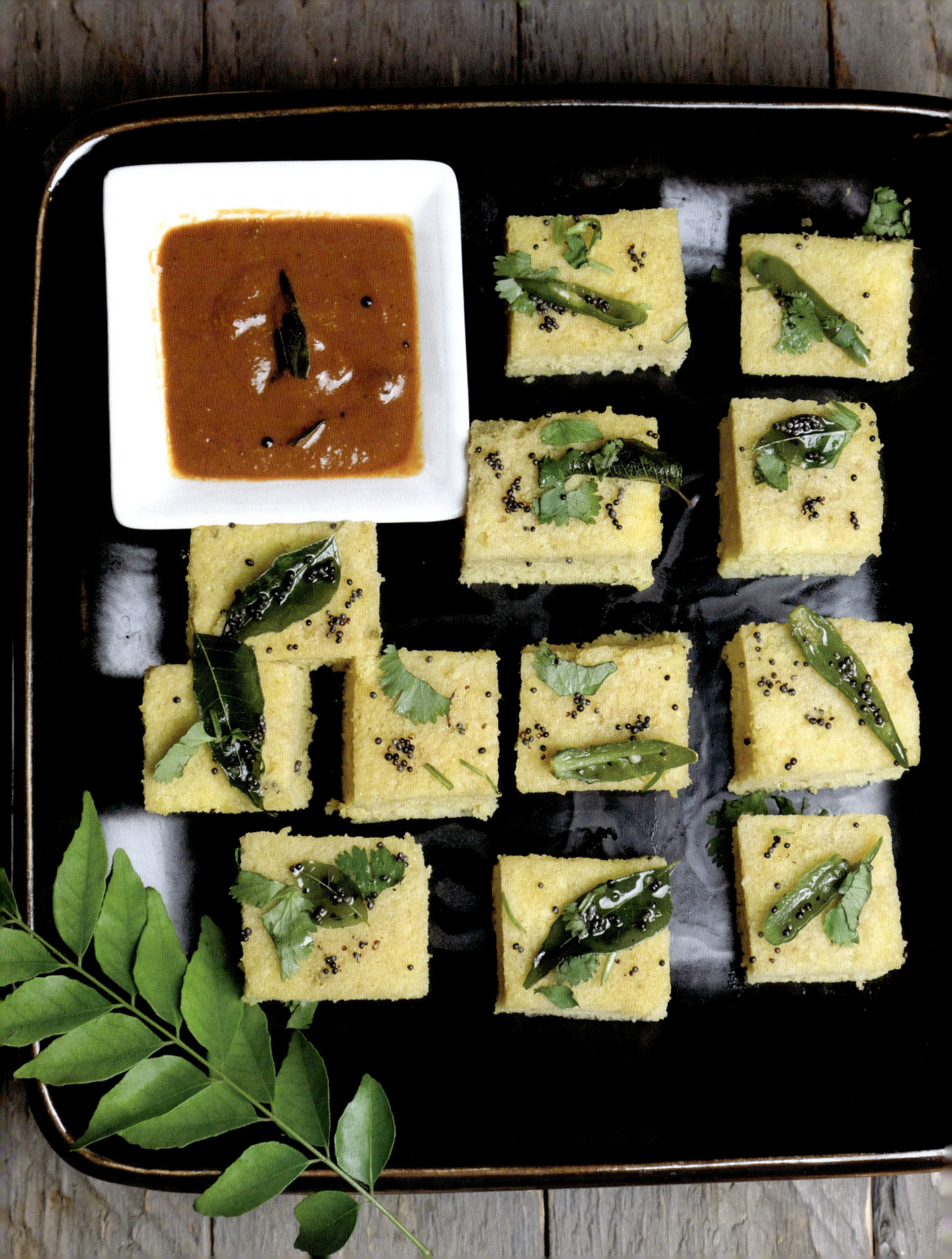

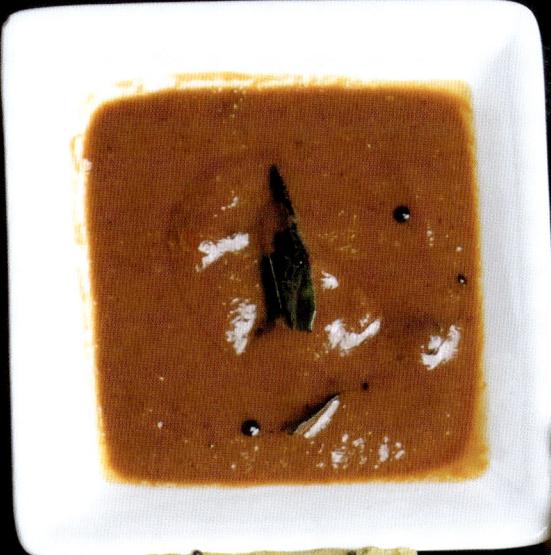

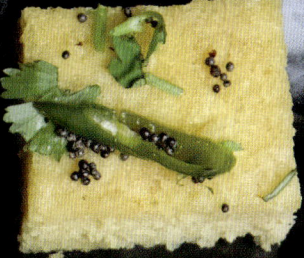

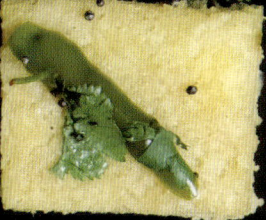

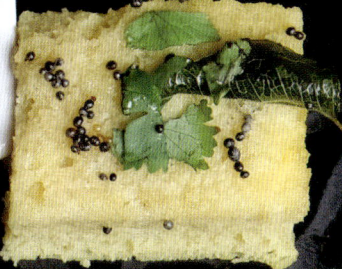

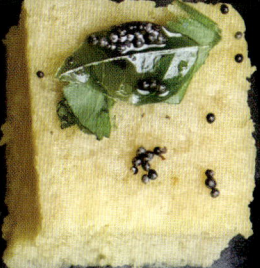

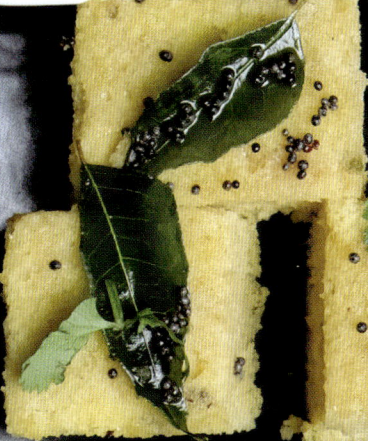

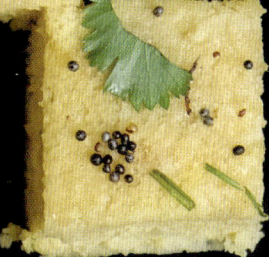

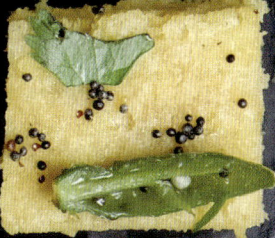

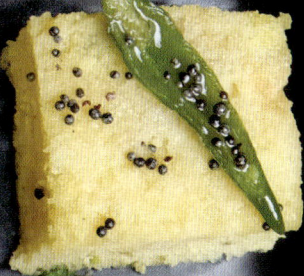

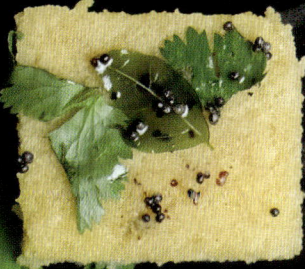

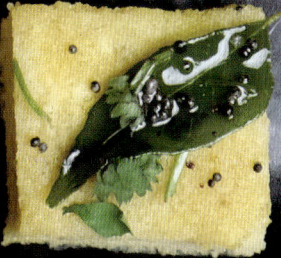

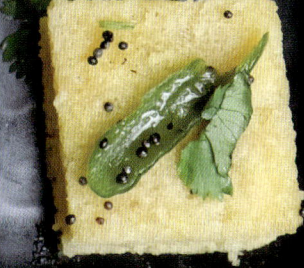

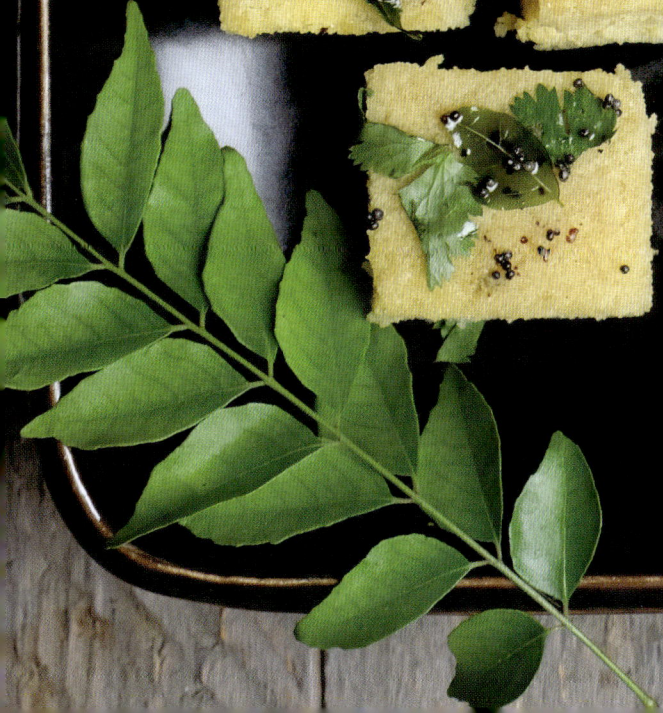

TAMARIND CHUTNEY

Ingredients

Tamarind: 2.5 oz (70 grams), about lemon sized

Oil: 2 tablespoons

Coriander seeds: 1 teaspoon

Cumin seeds: 1 teaspoon

White sesame: 1 tablespoon

Dry red chilis: 10

Jaggery: sufficient quantity

Garlic: 5 cloves (optional)

Salt: sufficient

Tempering ingredients

Mustard seeds: $1/8$ teaspoon

Black gram: $1/3$ teaspoon

Chickpea dal: $1/3$ teaspoon

Turmeric: $1/3$ teaspoon

Curry leaves: 2 stalks

Asafetida: ¼ teaspoon

Oil: 2 tablespoons

Directions

Soak the tamarind in hot water.

Heat oil in a frying pan and lightly fry the coriander seeds, cumin seeds, and white sesame seeds on a medium flame. Then add dry red chilis, garlic (optional) and continue frying for a short time. Grind all the above ingredients in a mixie, adding salt.

Add the soaked tamarind along with jaggery to the above mix in the mixie and grind them together, adding water to bring the chutney to a thin consistency.

Roast the tempering ingredients in oil in a frying pan. Then mix the tamarind chutney with the roasted tempering ingredients in the frying pan. Keep it in the pan for 5 minutes with the fire turned off. Now the mouth-watering tamarind chutney is ready to be enjoyed along with the delicious dhoklas.

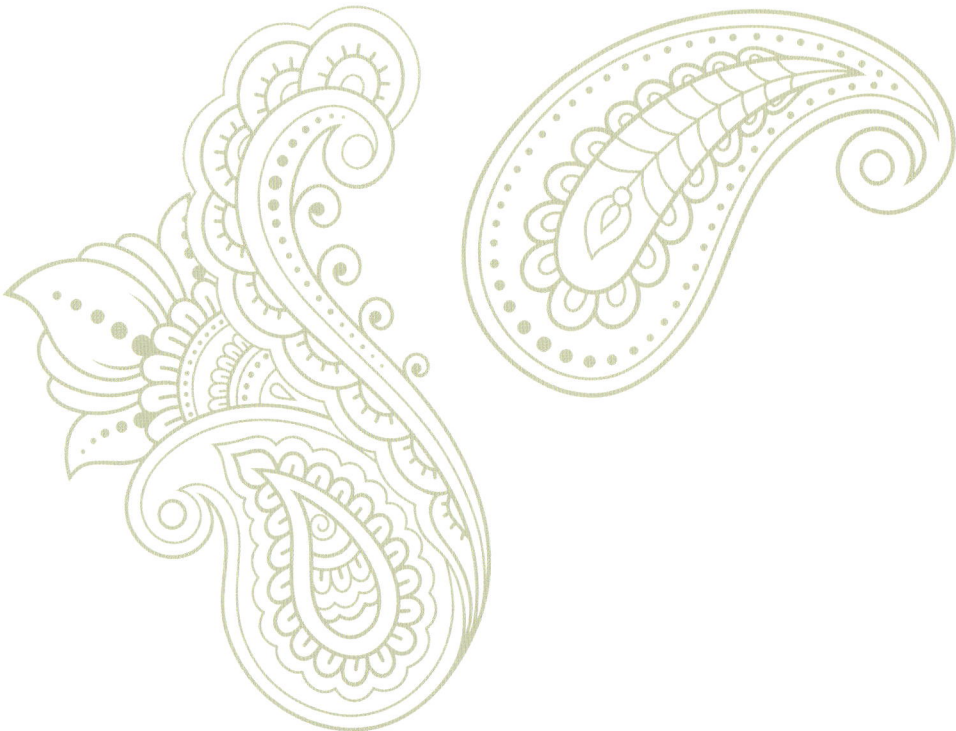

STEEL CUT OAT KICHIDI

Oat kichidi (also spelled khichdi), which is full of different vegetables and sprouts, is beneficial for Type 2 diabetics. It is usually eaten without chutney. However, I am giving you a recipe for a delicious green plantain curd chutney.

Ingredients

Oil: 2 tablespoons

Black gram: 1/8 teaspoon

Mustard seeds: 1/8 teaspoon

Cumin seeds: 1/8 teaspoon

Onion: 1, cut into pieces

Green chilis: 2, cut into pieces

Tomatoes: 2, cut into pieces

Carrots: 2, cut into pieces

Beans: 3 oz. (80 ml)

Green peas: 3 oz. (80 ml)

Sprouts: 6 oz. (160 ml) (optional)

Steel cut oats: 6 oz. (160 ml)

Ghee: 2 teaspoons

Turmeric powder: a pinch

Coriander leaves: small amount

Salt: sufficient quantity

Directions

Heat the oil in a saucepan, and fry the black gram, cumin seeds, and mustard seeds.

Add onion, green chilis, tomatoes, carrots and turmeric and cook on a medium flame for three minutes. Then add the sprouts (moong, chickpea, groundnut, etc.) and cook them for another three minutes.

Mix in the steel cut oats with the above cooked vegetables and sprouts, adding salt and 18 oz. (480 ml) of water. Cook the mixture for 50 minutes on a medium flame, covering the saucepan with a lid. Now and then, open the lid and stir the mixture. At the end, add ghee and some water if required.

Garnish the dish with coriander leaves, then serve with pleasure.

GREEN PLANTAIN CURD CHUTNEY

Ingredients

Green plantain: 1 (medium to large)

Curd (preferably sour): 12 oz. (320 ml)

Salt: sufficient quantity

Tempering ingredients

Mustard seeds: 1/8 teaspoon

Black gram: 1/3 teaspoon

Dry red chilis: 2

Curry leaves: 2 stalks

Asafetida: a pinch

Coriander leaves: 3 oz. (80 ml), chopped

Oil: 1 tablespoon

Directions

Roast the green plantain over a flame. After it cools down, peel it, remove the pulp and place it in a mixie. Grind it into the curd, adding salt. Take it out of the mixie and add another 6 oz. (160 ml) of curd to the mixture.

Temper the above curd paste with the tempering ingredients after frying them in oil.

Garnish the serving with coriander leaves.

BROWN RICE DOSA

Brown rice has a glycemic index of 50, and black gram, 43, making this dinner a highly recommended choice for Type 2 diabetics. Besides, this dosa-chutney combination is simply mouth-watering.

Ingredients

Brown rice: 12 oz. (320 ml)

Black gram husked: 6 oz. (160 ml)

Fenugreek seeds: ½ teaspoon

Salt: sufficient quantity

Directions

Soak the brown rice, black gram, and fenugreek seeds together for at least 8 hours. Then grind them together, adding water and salt, to a dosa batter consistency. Allow the batter to ferment for about 10 hours.

Using the batter, cook thin dosas in a pan using oil per your taste. You can make plain dosas, or dosas with onions and chilis cut into small pieces.

Serve with a tasty onion chutney.

. . . .

ONION CHUTNEY

Ingredients

Dry red chilis: 6

Onions(big): 2

Garlic: 6 cloves (optional)

Jaggery: small piece

Tamarind juice: 3 oz. (80 ml)

Salt: sufficient quantity

Oil: 1 tablespoon

Tempering ingredients

Oil: 2 tablespoons

Mustard seeds: 1/8 teaspoon

Cumin seeds: 1/8 teaspoon

Black gram: 1 teaspoon

Curry leaves: 2 stalks

Directions

Grind together the dry red chilis, onions, garlic cloves (optional), jaggery, tamarind juice, and salt to make the onion chutney.

Roast the tempering ingredients in oil and then mix in the onion chutney. Keep the chutney on a medium flame for two minutes to be ready to use.

GREEN GRAM PONGANALU

Green gram has a very low glycemic index of 31, and is rich in fiber and proteins, making it a good choice for Type 2 diabetics. This green gram dish with mustard chutney should not be missed. Note: Ponganalu are called paniyaram in Tamil, paddu in Kannada, and appe in Marathi.

Ingredients

Green gram (unhusked): 8 oz. (200 ml)

Salt: sufficient quantity

Ginger: 1 medium sized piece

Green chilis: 6

Carrots: 2, grated

Coriander leaves: half bunch, chopped

Baking soda: ¼ teaspoon

Turmeric powder: a pinch

Garam masala: ½ teaspoon

Lemon juice: 1 tablespoon

Oil: 3 tablespoons

Directions

Wash the green gram thoroughly and soak it in water for 10 hours. Then grind the green gram, adding salt, ginger, green chilis, and water to idli batter consistency.

Mix the grated carrots, chopped coriander leaves, baking soda, turmeric, garam masala, and lemon juice into the batter.

Using a pan with cavities, pour a little oil in each cavity, then add the batter. Close the pan with a lid and cook the ponganalu on a medium flame for 5 minutes. Then open the lid, flip the ponganalu, and cook them for another 3 to 4 minutes. This tempting dinner is ready.

The chutney to supplement the dish is mustard chutney.

MUSTARD CHUTNEY

Mustard seeds are a good source of several vitamins like vitamin C, and K, thiamine, riboflavin, vitamin B6, and folic acid, besides having antioxidant and anti-inflammatory properties.

Ingredients

Mustard seeds: 2 tablespoons

Curd, sour: 12 oz. (320 ml)

Turmeric powder: a pinch

Coriander leaves: small amount

Salt: sufficient quantity

Tempering ingredients

Ghee, oil: 1 tablespoon

Black gram: 1/3 teaspoon

Cumin seeds: 1/8 teaspoon

Dry red chilis: 1 cut into pieces

Asafetida: a pinch

Curry leaves: 2 stalks

Directions

Grind the mustard seeds in a small mixie jar or in a small traditional stone hand grinder (kalvam). Add a little water to make it into a paste.

Mix the curd into the paste, and add salt and turmeric powder.

Temper the chutney with the tempering ingredients after roasting them, preferably in ghee.

Garnish the mustard chutney with coriander leaves and this spicy dish is ready to give you a new feel when you enjoy it with the green gram dish.

INSTANT FINGER MILLET (RAGI) IDLI

Finger millet, whose helpfulness to diabetics has already been mentioned in the book, coupled with ajwain leaf curd chutney is one of the best choices for people with Type 2 diabetes.

Ingredients

Finger millet flour: 6 oz. (160 ml)
Upma rava (suji): 6 oz. (160 ml)
Curd, preferably sour: 12 oz. (320 ml)
Eno: 1 packet
Water: 3 oz. (80 ml)
Salt: sufficient quantity

Tempering ingredients

Ghee: 1 tablespoon
Mustard seeds: ¼ teaspoon
Chickpea dal: ½ teaspoon
Black gram: ½ teaspoon
Curry leaves: 2 stalks

Directions

Mix the finger millet flour and upma rava (suji) along with curd, salt, eno, and water to bring it to idli batter consistency. Set it aside for 15 minutes.

Temper the batter with the tempering ingredients after roasting them in ghee.

Using an idli cooker, cook the idlis for 10 to 15 minutes on a medium flame.

The chutney to go with these idlis is a marvelous ajwain leaf curd chutney.

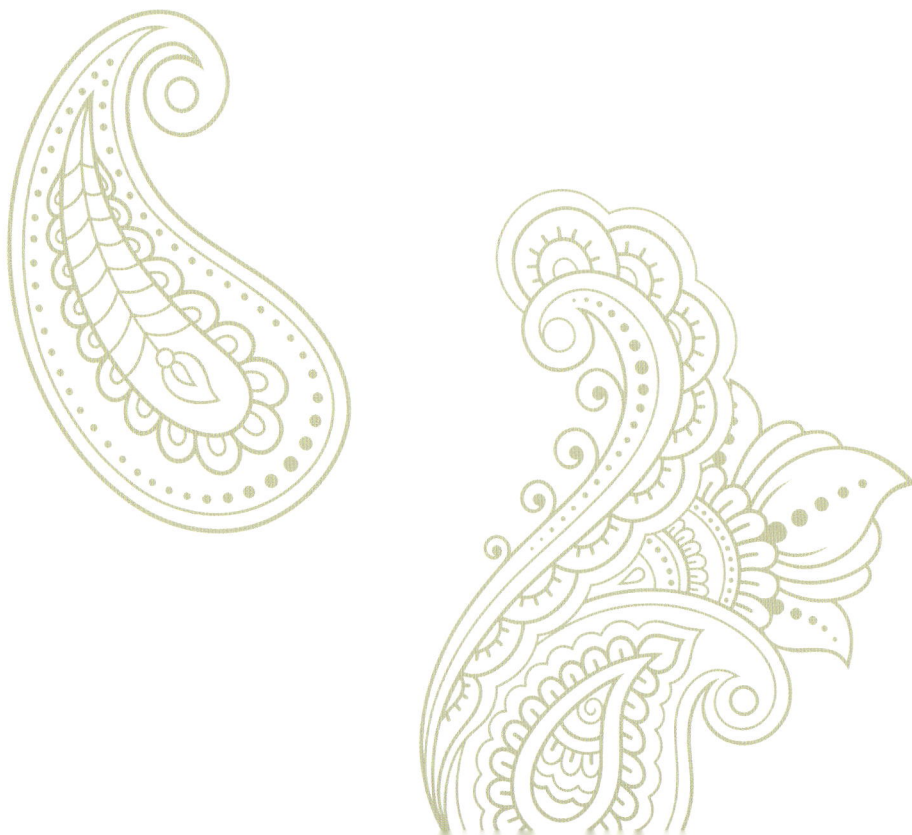

AJWAIN LEAF CURD CHUTNEY

Ajwain helps relieve indigestion, bloating, and gas. It has antifungal and antibacterial properties.

Ingredients

Ajwain leaves: 30

Cumin seeds: 1 teaspoon

Green chilis: 2

Curd, preferably sour: 12 oz. (320 ml)

Salt: sufficient quantity

Tempering ingredients

Chickpea dal: $1/3$ teaspoon

Black gram: $1/3$ teaspoon

Mustard seeds: $1/8$ teaspoon

Dry red chilis: 2

Curry leaves: 2 stalks

Asafetida: 1 pinch

Oil: 1 tablespoon

Directions

Cut the ajwain leaves into pieces and set them aside.

Grind cumin seeds and green chilis in a small mixie.

Then grind ajwain leaves coarsely without using water. Add sufficient salt.

Mix the ajwain leaf paste with the ground cumin-green chili paste.

Roast the tempering ingredients and mix them into the combined paste. Keep the mixture on the stove for 3 minutes after turning it off.

Mix the combined paste into the curd. Your yummy ajwain leaf curd chutney is ready to be enjoyed along with the ragi idlis.

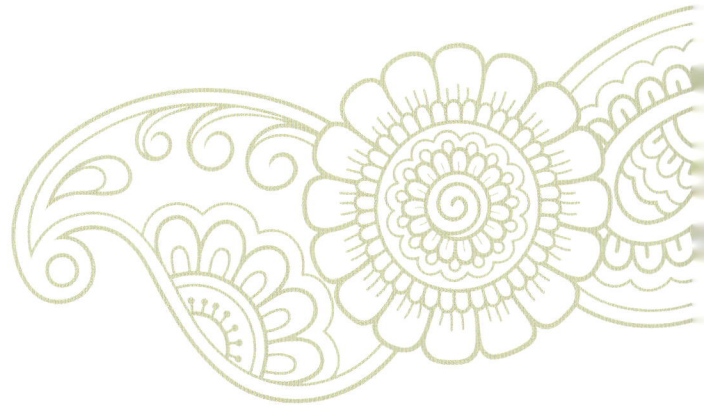

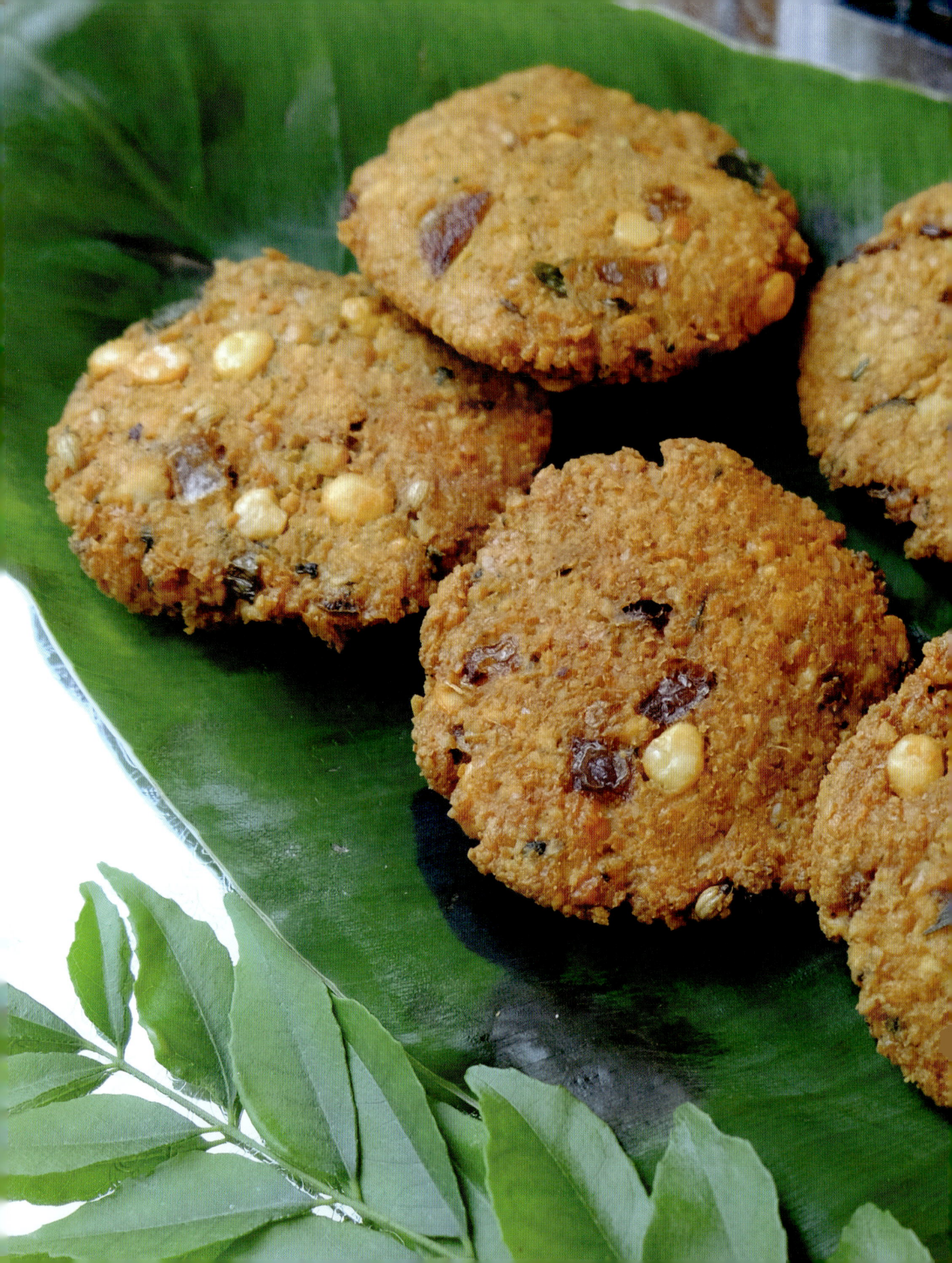

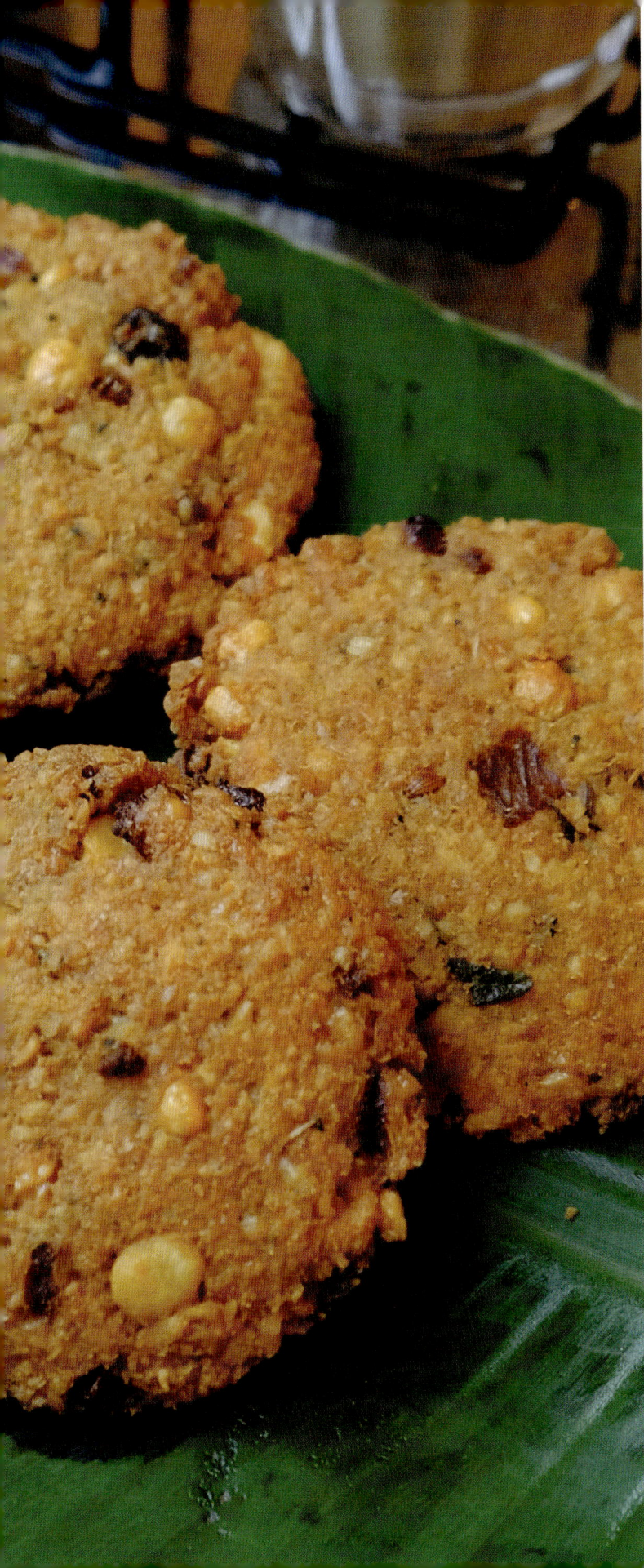

MOUTH-WATERING SNACKS

Masala Vada

TEMPERED KIDNEY BEANS

Kidney beans are rich in antioxidants, protein, and fiber, and with their small amount of carbohydrates, they are beneficial not only to people with diabetes but to all others.

Ingredients

Kidney beans: 12 oz. (320 ml)

Mustard seeds: ¼ teaspoon

Black gram: ½ teaspoon

Red chilis: 2, cut into pieces

Curry leaves: 2 stalks

Onions: 3 oz. (80 ml), chopped

Green chilis: 4, cut into pieces

Turmeric: a pinch

Salt: sufficient quantity

Oil: 1 tablespoon

Coriander leaves: a small bunch

Directions

Soak the kidney beans in water for 10 hours. Drain the water completely.

Heat the oil in a saucepan, and lightly roast the mustard seeds, black gram, and red chilis. Add the curry leaves and roast them further.

After all the ingredients are roasted, add the onions, green chilis, and turmeric, and cook the mixture for 3 minutes, covering the saucepan with a lid.

Then add the kidney beans and salt, and cook for 20 minutes on a medium flame, with the lid closed. Add water if necessary.

Garnish with the coriander leaves. This delicious kidney bean snack is ready for your relish.

TEMPERED CHICKPEAS

Chickpeas are high in fiber, vitamins, and various minerals along with offering plant-based protein. They have a low glycemic index, making them a good choice for people with Type 2 diabetes.

Ingredients

Oil: 1 tablespoon

Mustard seeds: ¼ teaspoon

Black gram: ½ teaspoon

Cumin seeds: ⅛ teaspoon

Asafetida: 1 pinch

Curry leaves: 2 stalks

Turmeric: a pinch

Onions: 3 oz. (80 ml), cut into pieces

Green chilis: 2

Chickpeas (unhusked): 6 oz. (160 ml)

Salt: sufficient quantity

Coriander leaves: small amount

Directions

Soak the chickpeas for 12 hours in water, then drain the water.

In a saucepan, lightly roast the mustard seeds, black gram, cumin seeds, and asafetida in oil. Then add the curry leaves and turmeric and continue roasting.

Once the above ingredients are fully roasted, add the onion, green chili, and salt, and cook for a few minutes, closing the saucepan with a lid.

Then add the chickpeas and 6 oz. (160 ml) of water. Cook the mixture on a low to medium flame for 20 minutes, covering the saucepan with a lid. You can add more water if required,

When chickpeas are ready, garnish the dish with coriander leaves and serve.

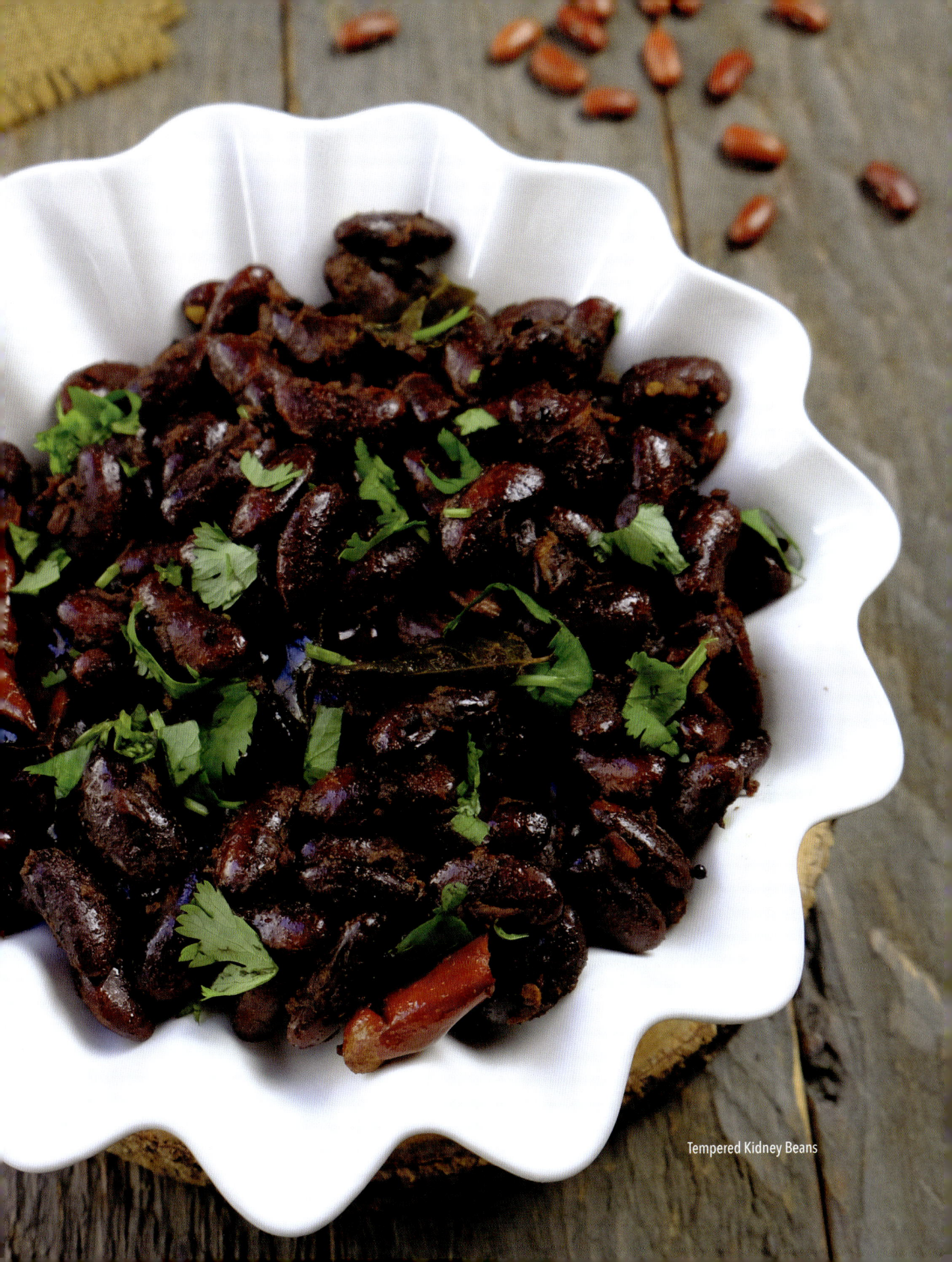

Tempered Kidney Beans

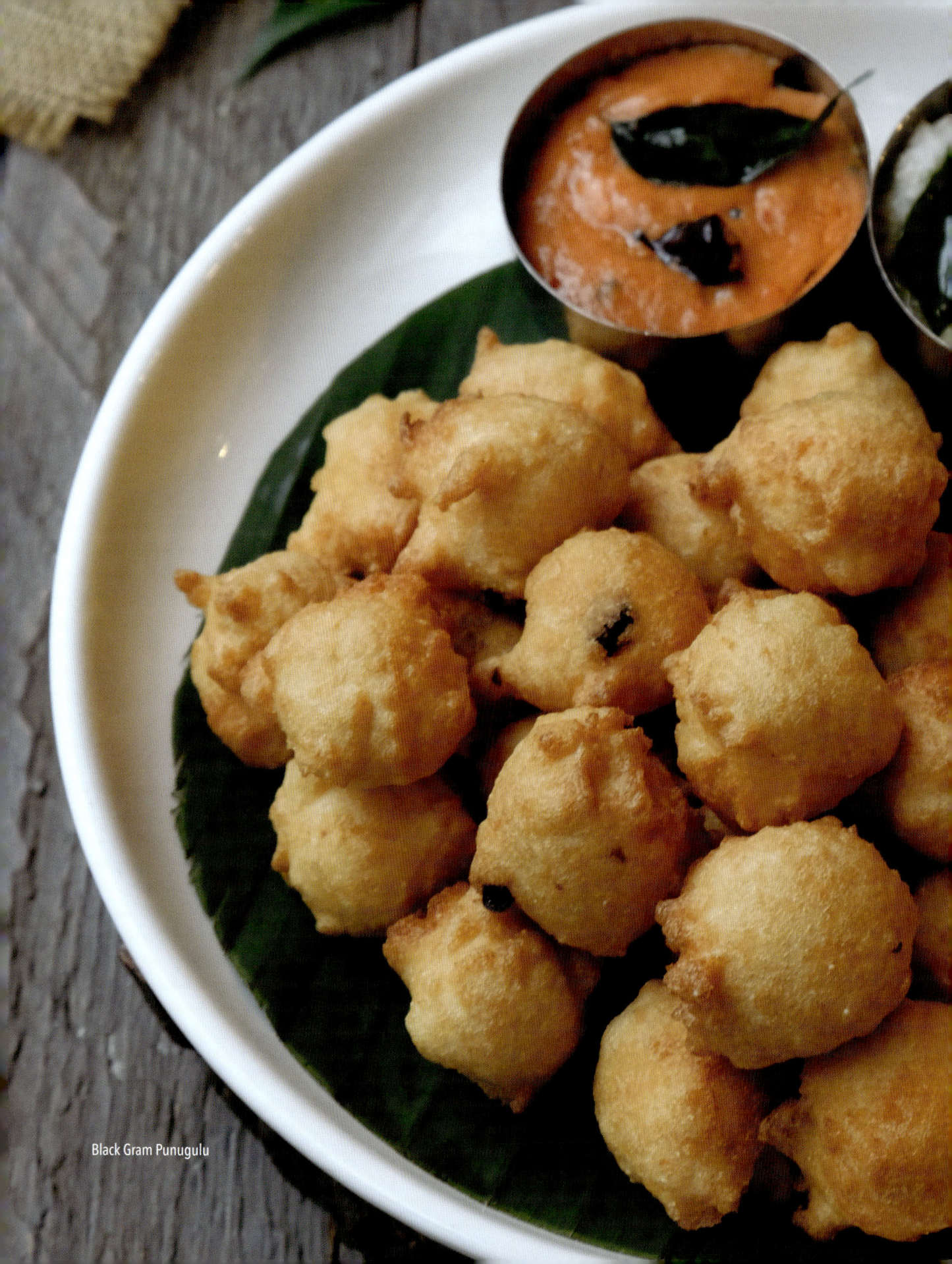
Black Gram Punugulu

BLACK GRAM PUNUGULU

Black gram is rich in minerals, vitamins, and proteins besides having a very low glycemic index.

Ingredients

Black gram (husked): 6 oz. (160 ml)

Jowar rawa: 1 teaspoon

Cumin seeds: teaspoon

Green chilis: 3

Onions: 3 oz. (80 ml), cut into pieces

Salt: sufficient quantity

Oil: 5 to 6 oz. (140 to 160 ml)

Directions

Soak the black gram for 8 hours in water, then grind it into a thick batter, adding a little water to a vada consistency.

Add the jowar rava, cumin seeds, green chilis, onions, and salt into the batter. Let the batter sit for 10 minutes.

Heat the oil in a frying pan. When it is hot, use the batter to make small lemon-sized balls, and fry them to a golden-brown color.

HORSE GRAM VADAS

Horse gram has a low glycemic index and is rich in fiber, proteins, vitamins, and iron, so it helps keep blood sugar levels low. It also has many properties that help promote digestive, heart, and brain health. It is highly recommended not only for people with diabetes but for anyone. It is also very delicious.

Ingredients

Horse gram: 6 oz. (160 ml)

Chickpea dal: 3 oz. (80 ml)

Garlic: 4 cloves

Ginger: a small piece

Green chilis: 6

Salt: sufficient quantity

Coriander leaves: a small quantity, chopped

Oil: 5 to 6 oz. (140 to 160 ml)

Directions

Wash the horse gram and soak it in water for 12 hours.

Soak the chickpea dal for 4 hours. Keep 1.5 oz. (40 ml) of chickpea dal aside.

Coarsely grind the horse gram dal and 1.5 oz. (40 ml) of chickpea dal together, without adding water. The batter should be thick enough for making vadas.

Grind the garlic (optional), ginger, and green chilis into a paste in a small mixie jar or a small stone hand grinder (kalvam). Mix the paste, salt, and the remaining 1.5 oz. (40 ml) of chickpea dal into the batter. Add chopped coriander leaves.

Heat the oil in a frying pan. Using both hands, make medium-sized round vadas, and fry them to a golden-brown color. Serve and enjoy.

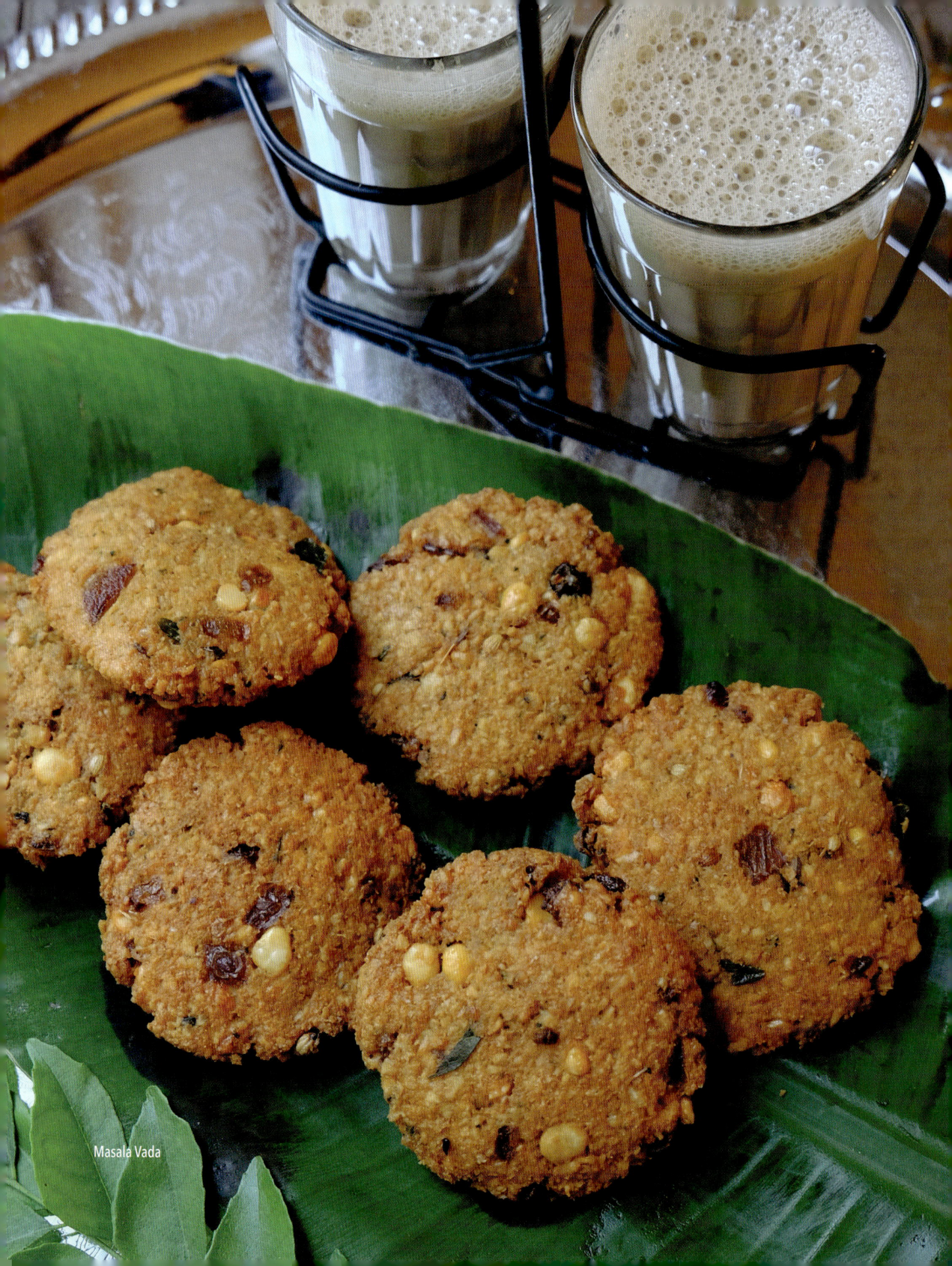

Masala Vada

MASALA VADA

Ingredients

Chickpea dal: 6 oz. (160 ml)

Ginger: a small piece

Garlic: 4 cloves (optional)

Rice flour: 1 teaspoon

Chickpea flour: 1 teaspoon

Cumin seeds: 1 teaspoon

Onions: 1.5 oz. (40 ml), cut into pieces

Green chilis: 3, cut into pieces

Coriander leaves: 1.5 oz. (40 ml)

Mint leaves: 1.5 oz. (40 ml)

Curry leaves: 1 stalk

Salt: sufficient quantity

Coriander seeds: 1/4 teaspoon

Garam masala: ¼ teaspoon

Oil: 5 to 6 oz. (140 to 160 ml)

Directions

Soak the chickpea dal in water for 4 hours.

Set aside a small handful of chickpea dal for a moment. To the remaining dal, add ginger and garlic (optional). Grind the mixture coarsely in a mixie, without adding water, to make a batter. Now mix the chickpea dal that was set aside into the batter.

Add the rice flour, chickpea flour, cumin seeds, onions, green chilis, coriander, mint and curry leaves, salt, coriander seeds and garam masala to the batter. If required, sprinkle no more than a tablespoon of water and mix it into the batter.

Using both your hands, make thin round small vadas from the batter. If the vadas are too thick, the batter inside will not be properly roasted.

Heat a saucepan with oil and place the vadas one by one into it. Roast them to a golden-brown color.

TEMPERED GREEN GRAM

Ingredients

Green gram (unhusked): 6 oz. (160 ml)

Oil: 2 tablespoons

Black gram: ½ teaspoon

Mustard seeds: ¼ teaspoon

Dry red chilis: 2, cut into pieces

Cumin seeds: ¼ teaspoon

Onions: 2 medium-sized, cut into pieces

Green chilis: 1

Ginger-garlic paste: 1 teaspoon

Dry red chili powder: ¼ teaspoon

Salt: sufficient quantity

Coriander leaves: 1.5 oz. (40 ml) for garnish

Directions

Wash the green gram thoroughly and soak it in water for two hours. Then cook it in a pressure cooker for one whistle only and set it aside. Add salt to taste.

Heat the oil in a frying pan and lightly fry the black gram, mustard seeds, dry red chilis, and cumin seeds. Add the onions and green chilis and continue frying.

After all these ingredients are sufficiently fried, add the ginger-garlic paste and fry it with the mixture.

Finally, add the boiled green gram, mixing it thoroughly with all the above ingredients and some water. Cook the mixture for a few minutes, then add the dry red chili powder. Keep it on the stove until all the water fully evaporates.

Garnish with coriander leaves and serve.

AJWAIN LEAF BAJJI

Ajwain helps relieve indigestion, bloating, and gas. It has antifungal and antibacterial properties. When ragi is coupled with ajwain, it makes an excellent meal for people with Type 2 diabetes.

Ingredients

Ajwain leaves: 15

Chickpea flour: 6 oz. (160 ml)

Salt: sufficient quantity

Dry red chili powder: ¼ teaspoon

Turmeric powder: a pinch

Garam masala: ¼ teaspoon

Baking soda: a pinch

Oil: 5 to 6 oz. (140 to 160 ml)

Directions

Add all the ingredients listed, except ajwain leaves and oil, to the chickpea flour. Add water little by little to make a batter with the consistency of bajji.

Now take the washed ajwain leaves one by one, then dip them in the batter and fry them in oil to a golden-brown color.

REJUVENATING BOILED PEANUT SNACK

Groundnuts (peanuts) have a low glycemic index and are rich in healthy fats that help reduce bad cholesterol. They are also known to improve memory, prevent various types of cancer, reduce weight, and maintain blood sugar levels. Green gram and chickpeas contain less amount of carbohydrates and also have a low glycemic index. This snack is thus a good choice for people with Type 2 diabetes

Ingredients

Peanuts: 3 oz. (80 ml)

Green gram: 1.5 oz. (40 ml)

Chickpeas: 1.5 oz. (40 ml)

Honey: 2 teaspoons

Lemon juice: 1 tablespoon

Salt: a sufficient quantity

Tempering ingredients

Black gram: ½ teaspoon

Mustard seeds: ¼ teaspoon

Dry red chilis: 2

Green chilis: 2

Grated ginger: 1 tablespoon

Curry leaves: 2 stalks

Ghee: 1 tablespoon

Directions

Soak the peanuts, green gram, and chickpeas in water for 12 hours. Drain the water.

Cook the above three items in 12 oz. (320 ml) of water in a pressure cooker to one whistle. Drain any residual water and add lemon juice, honey, and salt.

Temper the preparation with the tempering ingredients after roasting them in ghee. This amazing strength-giving snack is ready for your relish.

BETEL LEAF BAJJI

Betel leaf has antioxidant, anti-inflammatory, and antimicrobial properties. It helps in digestion and is known to control blood sugar levels. Betel leaf bajji is one of the best choices for people with Type 2 diabetics.

Ingredients

Chickpea flour: 6 oz. (160 ml)

Rice flour: 1 teaspoon

Salt: sufficient quantity

Turmeric: a pinch

Dry red chili powder: ¼ teaspoon

Oil: 4 oz. (150 ml)

Betel leaves: 15

Directions

Put the chickpea flour and rice flour in a saucepan. Add 3 oz. (80 ml) of water, salt, turmeric, and dry red chili powder to make a semi-thick batter. If required, add more water.

Heat the oil in a saucepan. When it is fully hot, dip the betel leaves one by one in the chickpea batter, and place them gently in the hot oil. It is advisable to fry only 3 at a time. After they are well roasted, put them in a large colander set on a plate where the leaves can drip dry.

CORIANDER LEAF PAKODI (PAKORA)

Coriander leaves are a source of vitamin C, calcium, magnesium, potassium, and iron. They are known to lower blood sugar and blood pressure, fight infections, and promote brain, heart, skin, kidney and digestive health, making coriander pakodi a highly preferred snack for people with Type 2 diabetes.

Ingredients

Coriander leaves: 12 oz. (320 ml), chopped

Chickpea flour: 6 oz. (160 ml)

Rice flour: 1 teaspoon

Green chilis: 4

Salt: sufficient quantity

Turmeric: a pinch

Oil: 4 oz. (150 ml)

Directions

Wash the chopped coriander leaves and place them in a bowl. Add chickpea flour, rice flour, chopped green chilis, salt, and turmeric. Then, mixing with water, stir the ingredients into a semi-thick paste.

Heat the oil in a frying pan. After the oil is fully hot, slowly place pebble-sized lumps in it and roast them sufficiently till they are ready to serve.

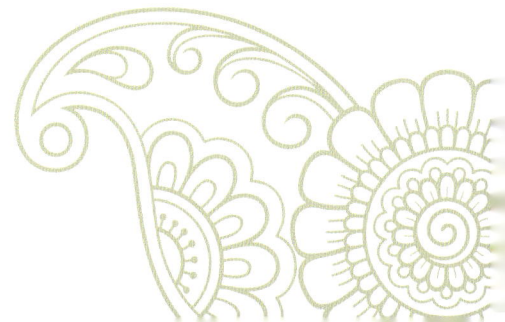

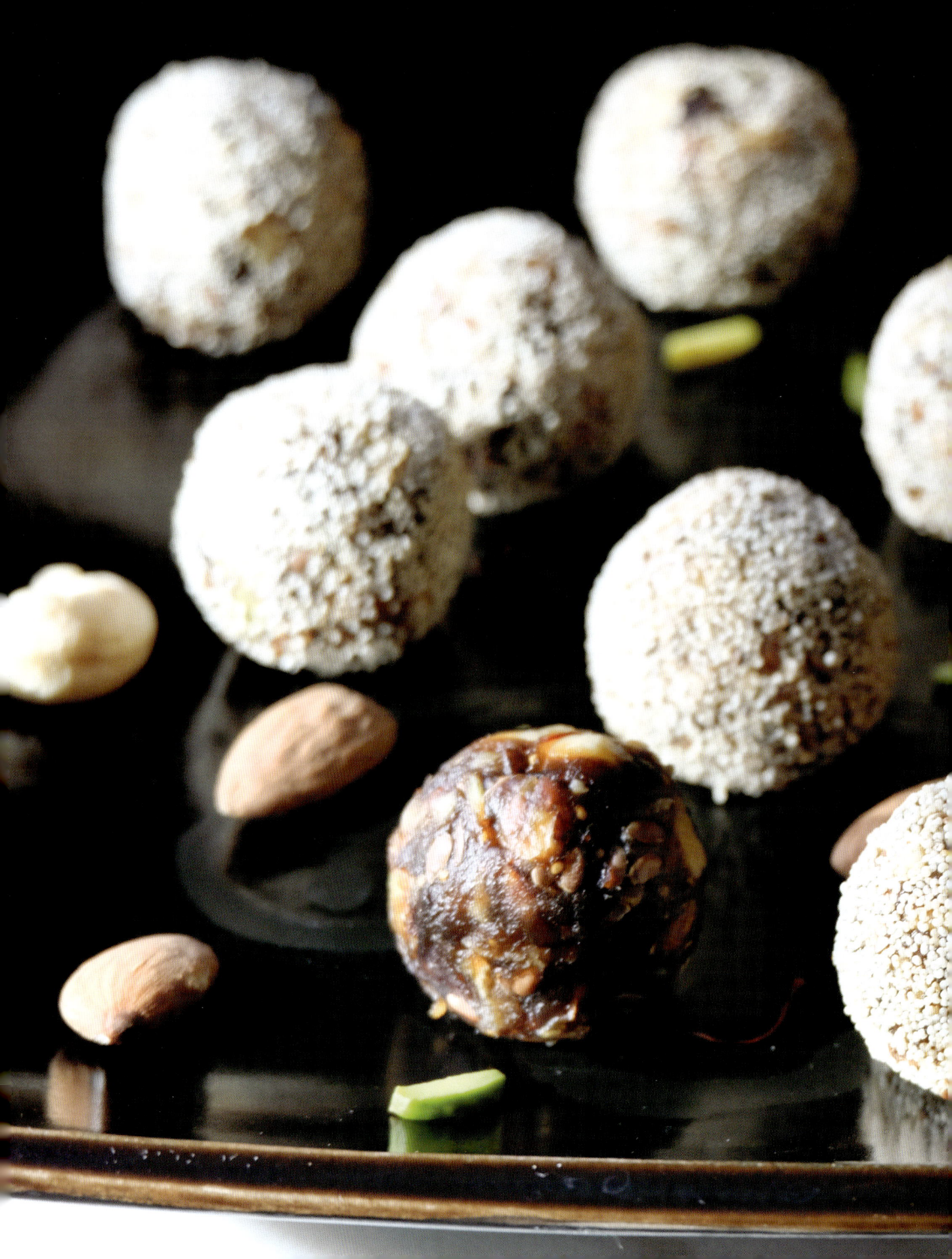

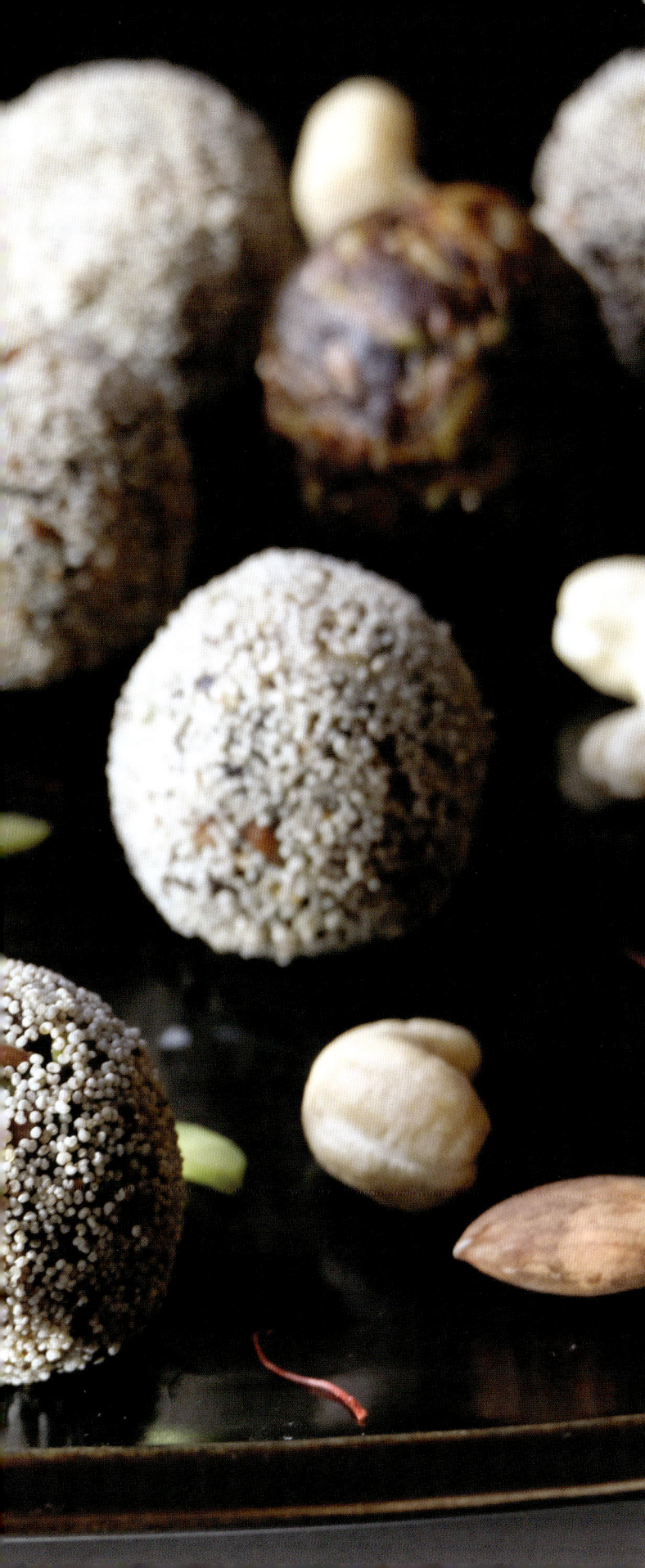

SAVORY SWEETS

Dry Fruit Laddu

Since I have shown you different recipes for your breakfast, lunch, and dinner as well as snacks that are mostly free from grains and grain flour, your carbohydrate intake will definitely be less than normal. This allows you to happily indulge in some sweets. Some of the sweets I suggest are made only with fruit, and some with jaggery. Both of these are better than white sugar for people with diabetes. In fact, you can happily eat sweets, of course in a limited quantity, made with sugar also as I have already told you. However, sweets should be eaten in moderation only, i.e., twice or thrice a week is enough to give you some taste enjoyment without causing you any harm.

CARROT HALWA

Carrot is rich in fiber, antioxidants, nutrients, and vitamins. It not only helps in digestion but also in controlling blood sugar levels. People with Type 2 diabetes can happily enjoy this sweet.

Ingredients

Cashew nuts: 9
Carrot: 18 oz. (480 ml), grated
Jaggery: 3 oz. (80 ml), grated
Date fruit paste: 6 oz. (160 ml)
Cardamom powder: ½ teaspoon
Ghee: 3 tablespoons

Directions

Roast the cashew nuts in ghee to a golden-brown color and set them aside.

Mix the grated carrot with the jaggery in a saucepan and cook it for 30 minutes on a low flame, sprinkling in a little water. When the mixture is cooked, it turns into a gummy jaggery paste.

Add the date fruit paste and cardamom powder to the paste. Take a plate and apply ghee all over the surface. Place some carrot halwa on it. Garnish it with cashew nuts and it's ready to serve.

BLACK GRAM (URAD DAL) LADDU

Black gram laddus, called sunnundalu in Telugu and karuppu ulundu in Tamil, are noted for their invigorating properties and making the body strong and healthy. You can increase the quantity of jaggery if you like the laddus to be sweeter.

Ingredients

Black gram (husked): 12 oz. (320 ml)
Jaggery: 9 oz. (240 ml)
Ghee: 6 oz. (160 ml)

Directions

Roast the black gram to a golden-brown color. After it cools down, grind it into a fine powder.

Grind the jaggery and mix it into the black gram flour. Then slowly adding ghee, make laddus with the black gram jaggery mixture.

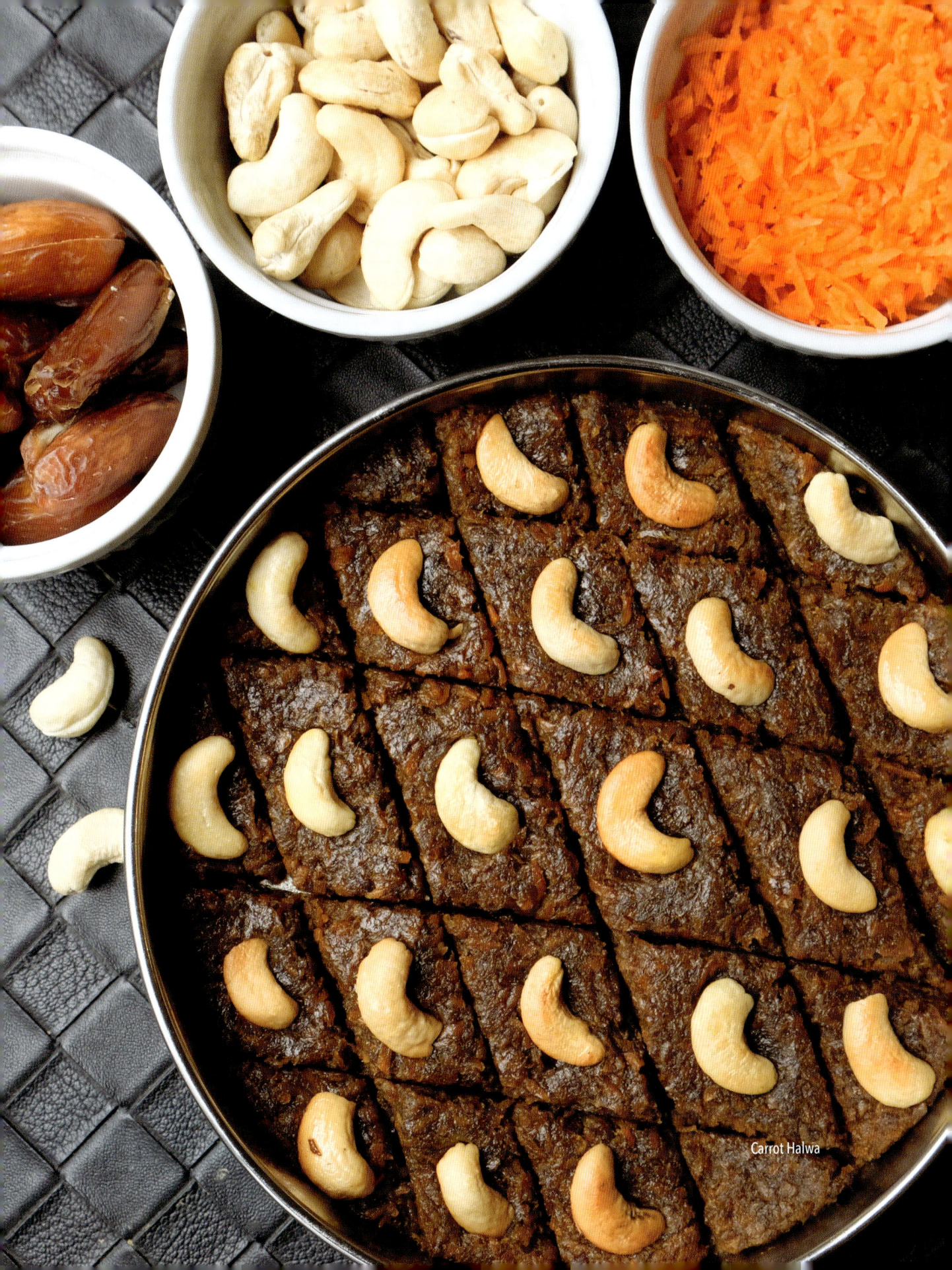

Carrot Halwa

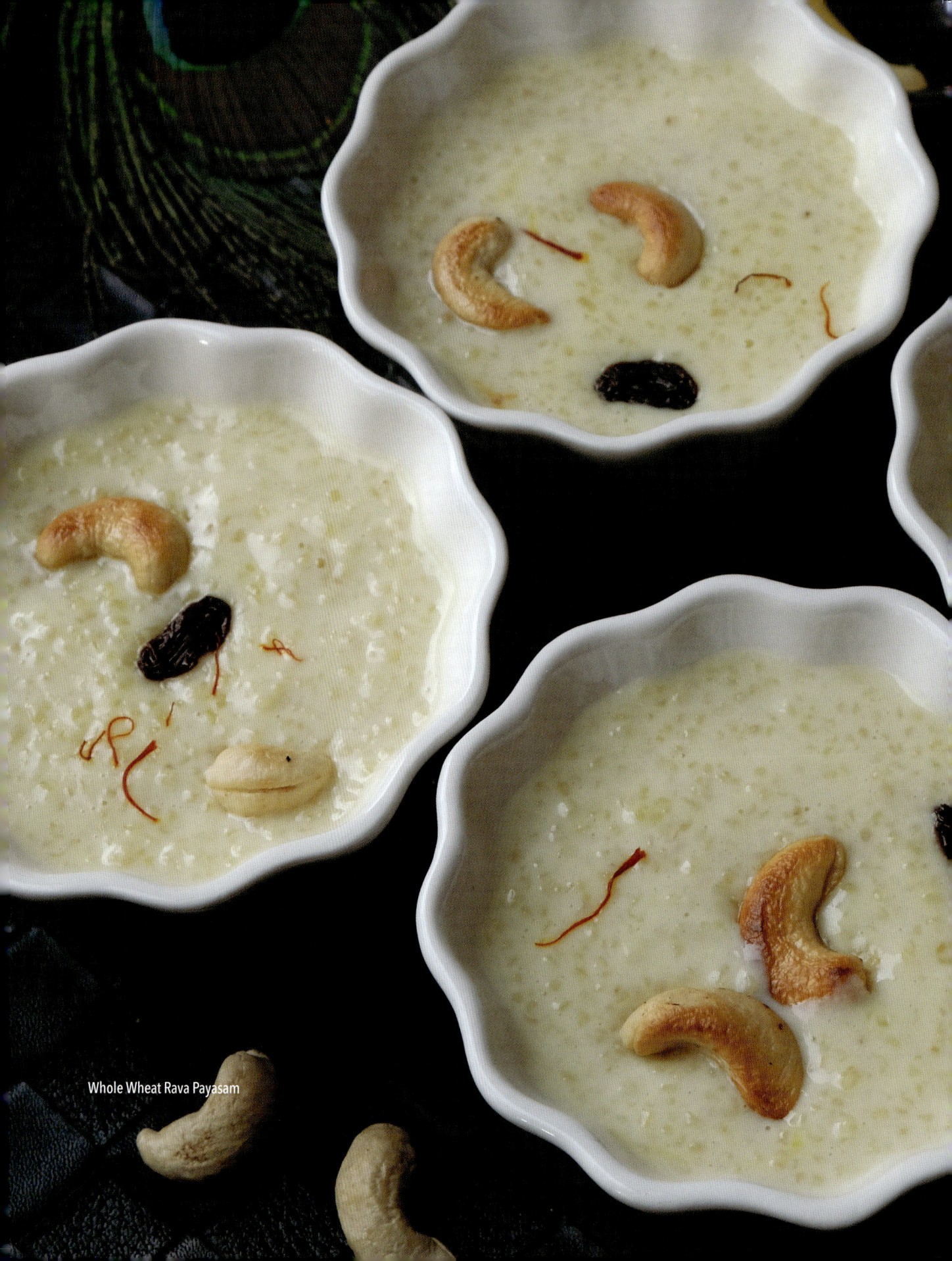
Whole Wheat Rava Payasam

WHOLE WHEAT RAVA PAYASAM

Whole wheat rava has a low glycemic index (47), and is rich in fiber, vitamins, nutrients, minerals, and antioxidants. Since you have cut down your carbohydrate intake, you can happily enjoy this sweet even though it is made with sugar.

Ingredients

Ghee: 3 tablespoons

Cashew nuts: 3 oz. (80 ml)

Raisins: 4 teaspoons

Whole wheat rava: 3 oz. (80 ml)

Milk: 24 oz. (640 ml)

Sugar: 4.5 oz (120 ml)

Saffron: a pinch (optional)

Cardamom powder: ½ teaspoon

Directions

Pour ghee in a saucepan and fry the cashews. In the final stages of frying, add raisins and fry them. Set aside.

Boil the whole wheat rava in 9 oz. (240 ml) of water. After it is softly cooked, add milk and continue cooking the whole wheat rava for 10 minutes more.

Add sugar, saffron, cardamom powder to the fried cashews and raisins. Fry them again on a low flame for two minutes, stirring with a cooking spoon. Then add this mixture to the whole wheat rava. If required, add some water to bring the payasam to the required consistency.

Turn off the stove and keep the mixture there for two minutes. Your whole wheat rava payasam is now ready to give you a delightful taste.

BEETROOT LADDU

Beetroot is high in fiber and low in carbohydrates, so it helps control blood sugar levels. It is also rich in antioxidants and many nutrients.

Ingredients

Cashews, almonds and raisins: 3 oz. (80 ml)

Ghee. 3 tablespoons

Beetroot grated: 18 oz. (480 ml)

Jaggery grated: 3 oz. (80 ml)

Cardamom powder: ½ teaspoon

Directions

Roast cashews, almonds, and raisins to golden-brown color in a tablespoon of ghee. Set it aside.

Roast the grated beetroot in two tablespoons of ghee, until it is no longer raw. Add jaggery and cook it on a medium flame, constantly stirring it with a cooking spoon until it becomes sticky.Add cardamom powder and the roasted cashews, almonds, and raisins.

Applying ghee to your palms, make the mixture into medium-sized round laddus.

DRY FRUIT LADDU

The ingredients in the dry fruit laddu are rich in nutrients like potassium, iron, calcium and magnesium, which can help boost your immunity. They are also rich in dietary fiber. Moreover, the natural sweetness in the laddu can help satisfy your cravings for sweets without causing a spike in blood sugar levels.

Ingredients

Almonds: 10, thinly cut

Cashew nuts: 10, thinly cut

Acrots: 2, thinly cut

Pistas: 10, thinly cut

Dry coconut: 2 tablespoons, grated

Pumpkin seeds: 2 teaspoons

Ghee: 2 tablespoons

Anjuras: 2, cut into pieces

Dates: 6 oz. (160 ml) seedless

Raisins: 1 tablespoon

Flax seeds: 1 teaspoon

Saffron: ½ teaspoon

Cardamom powder: ½ teaspoon

Poppy seeds: 1 teaspoons

Directions

Roast the almonds, cashews, acrots, pistas, dry coconut, and pumpkin seeds in ghee to a golden-brown color.

In another saucepan, combine anjura, dates, and raisins. Add four or five teaspoons of water and cook them for five minutes.

Mix the roasted and cooked ingredients, adding the flax seeds, saffron, and cardamom powder. Make small, round laddus. Roll the dry fruit laddus on a plate with poppy seeds so that the poppy seeds stick to the laddus, providing a delicious taste and texture.

SESAME PEANUT LADDU

The nutritional content of sesame and peanut help keep the body healthy, active, and strong.

Ingredients

White sesame seeds: 6 oz. (160 ml)

Peanuts: 6 oz. (160 ml)

Jaggery: 9 oz. (240 ml), grated

Cardamom powder: ¼ teaspoon

Directions

Roast the sesame seeds and peanuts separately. Then grind the seeds and roasted peanuts separately into smooth powders.

Mix both the powders together with jaggery and grind them again.

Transfer the mixture to a bowl and add ¼ teaspoon of cardamom powder.

Make medium-sized laddus from the mixture. No ghee is needed in the process as the sesame seed powder is internally oily and jaggery is sticky. If you want the laddus to be sweeter, you can add more jaggery.

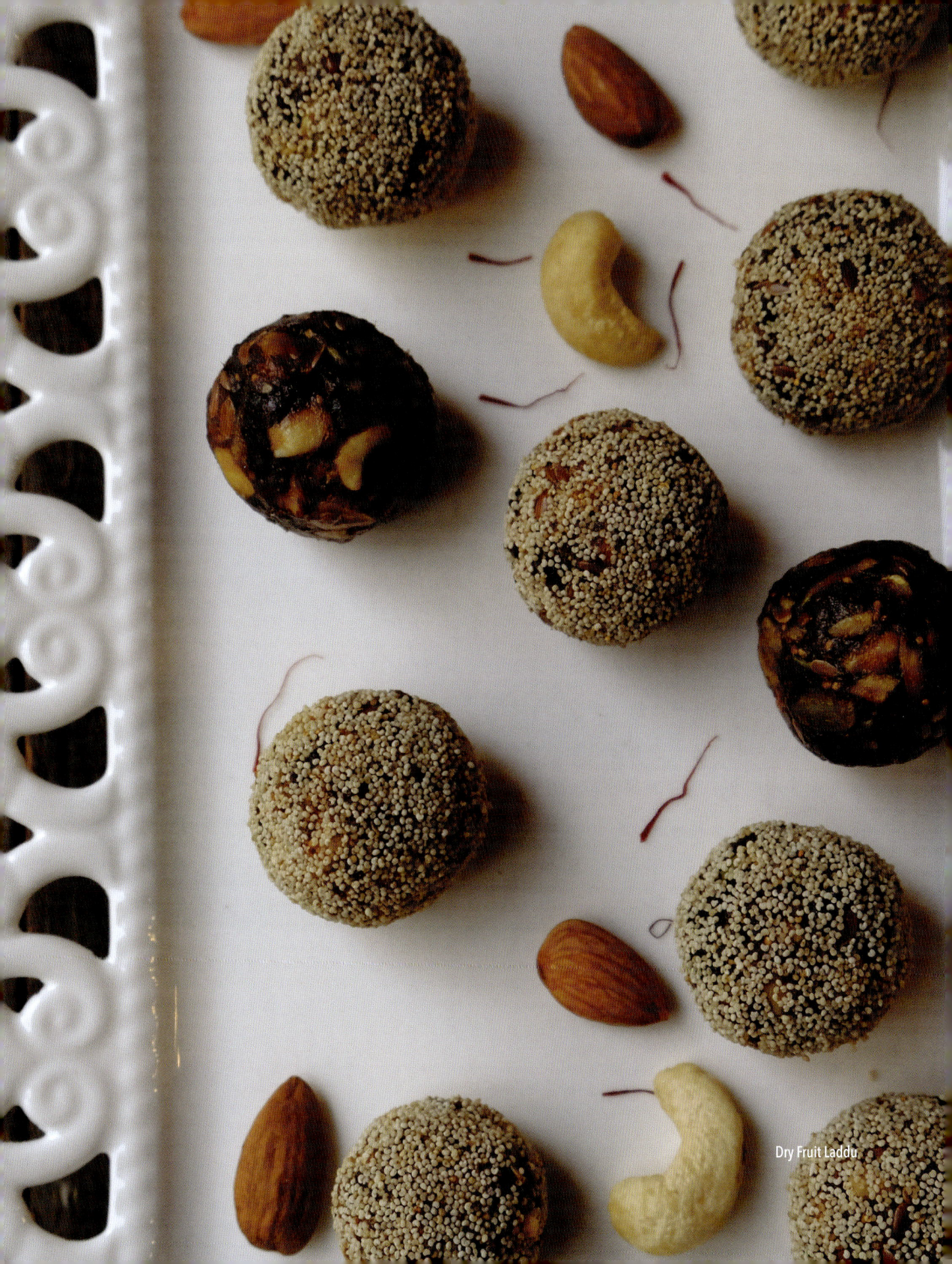

Dry Fruit Laddu.

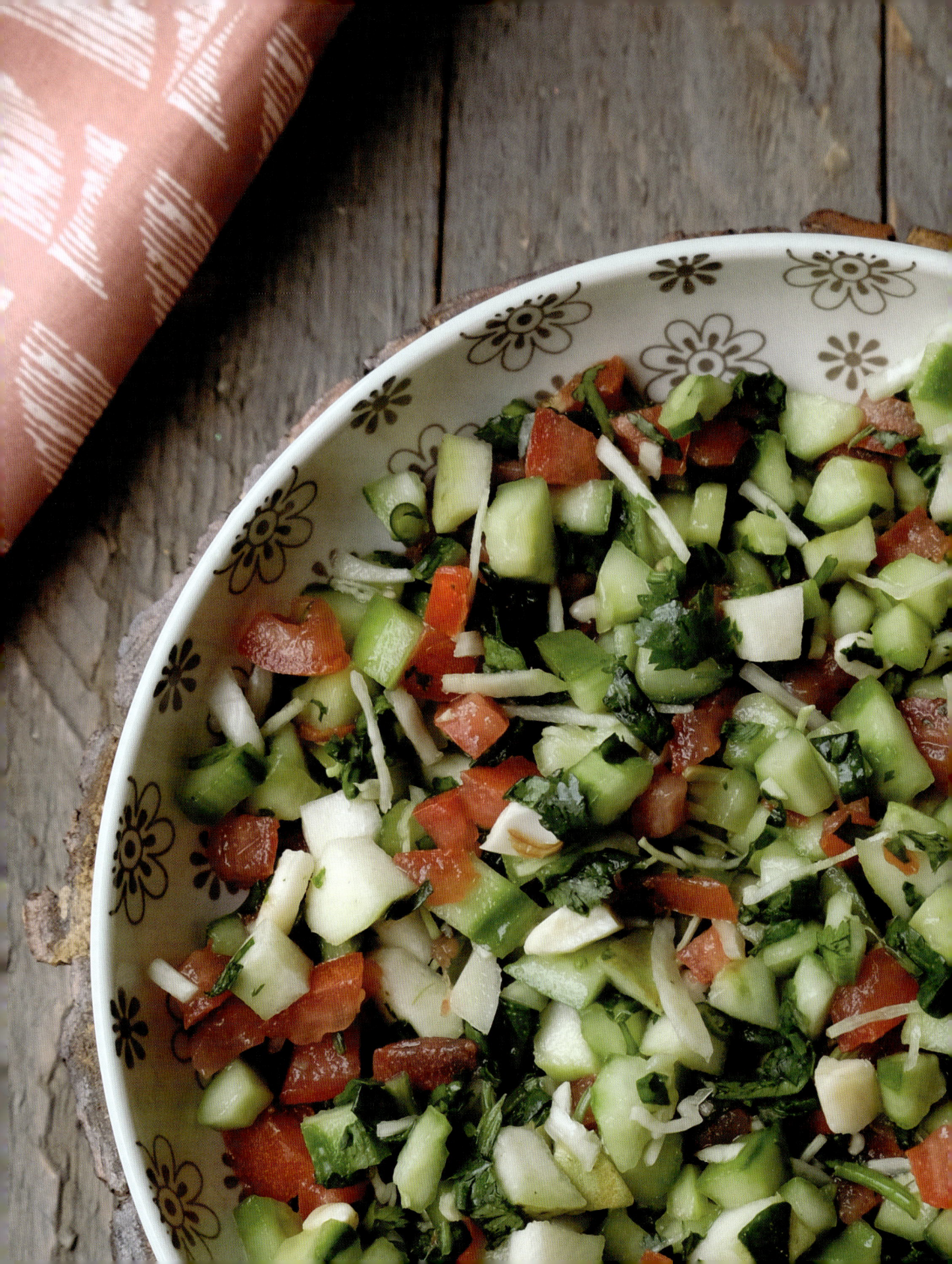

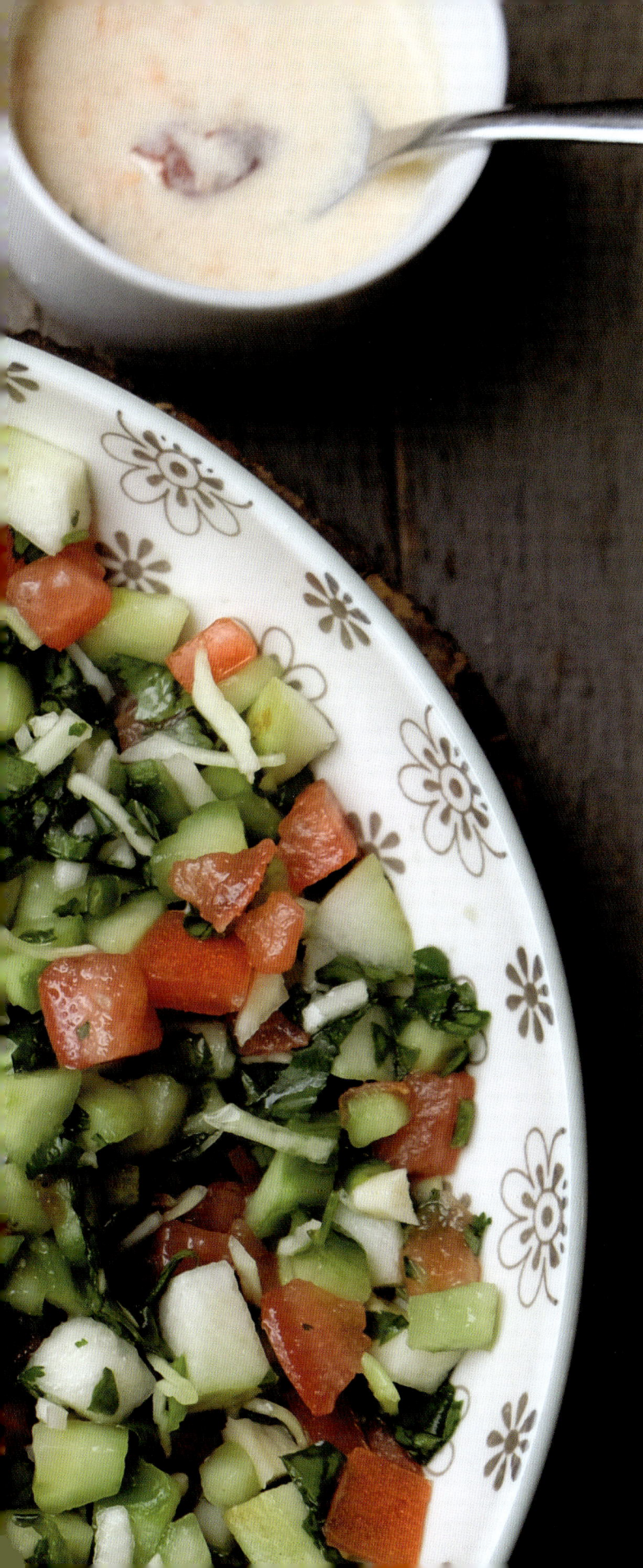

SUPER-TASTY INDIAN SALADS

SUCCULENT TRADITIONAL DRESSINGS

Tomato Ridge Gourd Salad

Making Super-Tasty Salads

Salads contain raw vegetables, fruits, leafy vegetables, sprouts, nuts, and seeds. They are normally eaten with a dressing to make them more delicious. An Indian traditional dressing may be spicy, sour, or sweet and salty, and is often made with vegetables ground into a thin paste, along with lemon juice, ground chilis, honey, and salt. The dressings are often a thick liquid or a semisolid substance.

Here are ingredients you can use to make salads:

- **Vegetables:** Carrots, beetroots, radishes, tomatoes, onions, ridge gourd, cucumber, capsicum, gooseberry, green chilis, coconut, or any other vegetable pleasing to your taste.

- **Leafy vegetables:** Spinach, mint, coriander, young tamarind leaves, chickpea leaves, betel leaves, drumstick leaves, curry leaves, and any other edible leafy vegetable.

- **Fruits:** Apples, grapes, watermelon, cantaloupe, guava, pomegranate, banana, papaya, green mangoes, ripe mangoes, jackfruit, chikoo, pineapple, or any other fruit you enjoy eating.

- **Nuts and lentils:** Almonds, cashew, walnuts, boiled ground nuts, and various other peas and lentils.

- **Sprouts and Microgreens:** Sprouts are produced from germinating peas and lentils like peanuts, green gram, black gram, chickpea, pigeon pea (toor dal), etc. in 3 to 5 days, while microgreens are greens that have been harvested between 7 and 14 days. Microgreens can also be produced from very small seeds in your kitchen, such as mustard seeds, cumin, ajwain, coriander seeds, fenugreek seeds, and sorghum, ragi, millets, horse gram, sesame as well as the seeds of different leafy vegetables.

Sprout Your Own Peas and Lentils

Take the peas and lentils of your choice, wash them thoroughly and soak them in water for 10 hours. Then drain the water and wrap them in a clean, thin cloth. Wash them in water daily, then rinse them and wrap them back in the cloth until they sprout. It may take four or five days for them to germinate. After germination, they can be used in salads.

Microgreens Are Easy to Produce

Sow seeds of your choice in your yard, water them, and wait for 10 to 15 days when the first set of leaves appear. Cut them close to the surface and consume them. Microgreens can also be grown in your house, in trays with clay, and exposed to sunlight.

Sprouts and microgreens are rich in minerals, vitamins, fiber, antioxidants, anti-carcinogens and anti-aging elements. They contain less carbohydrates and more plant-based proteins. Sprouts and microgreens, if consumed often, not only control blood sugar but also help preserve good health.

The Importance of Salad Dressings in Your Diet

Many people indulge in eating heavy meals, full of carbohydrates, and end up with chronic diseases—especially Type 2 diabetes—and dedicating their lives to medicines. So how can someone who is used to eating sumptuous meals get accustomed to eating foods consisting of raw vegetables? This is a question confronting most of us.

To make salads as tasty as your usual heavy dinners, I suggest you make delicious dressings to go with the salads. In most Western countries, dressings are made in factories, and people purchase them pre-made. But since your health is in your hands, it is far better to prepare dressings with fresh ingredients yourself.

In this section, I will introduce you to 7 dressings that are unbelievably tasty to complement any salad.

Note: All these salads can be prepared even if some of the ingredients are not available; neither the preparation nor the taste will be affected.

SALADS

SPROUT SALAD

Ingredients

Green gram sprouts: 1.5 oz. (40 ml)

Black eyed beans: 1.5 oz. (40 ml)

Chickpeas: 1.5 oz. (40 ml)

Grated cabbage: 1.5 oz. (40 ml)

Tomato: 6 oz. (160 ml), cut into pieces

Cucumber: 6 oz. (160 ml), cut into pieces

Grated carrot: 1.5 oz. (40 ml)

Honey: 1 tablespoon

Cashew nuts: 3 oz. (80 ml), chopped

Pepper powder: 1 teaspoon

Oil: 1 tablespoon

Salt: sufficient quantity

Directions

Wash all the vegetables thoroughly in salt water to cleanse them, then chop them. Next, put all the vegetables into a bowl. Mix them well and add honey, oil, and salt.

Enjoy this salad by slowly chewing the vegetables along with any of the seven dressings, as per your taste. However, I suggest you enjoy this salad with the coconut milk dressing.

FRUIT SALAD

Ingredients

Sprouted green gram: 3 oz. (80 ml)

Grated carrot: 1.5 oz. (40 ml)

Soaked groundnuts: 1.5 oz. (40 ml)

Apple: 3 oz. (80 ml), cut into pieces

Pomegranate seeds: 3 oz. (80 ml)

Papaya fruit: 3 oz. (80 ml), cut into pieces

Grapes: 15

Raisins: 10

Split cashews: 10

Orange: 5 segments

Sunflower seeds: 1 tablespoon

Directions

Put all the ingredients into a bowl and mix thoroughly. Top it with any of the seven dressings and eat the salad, slowly chewing it and enjoying its taste. I suggest the yellow cucumber curd dressing to go along with this salad.

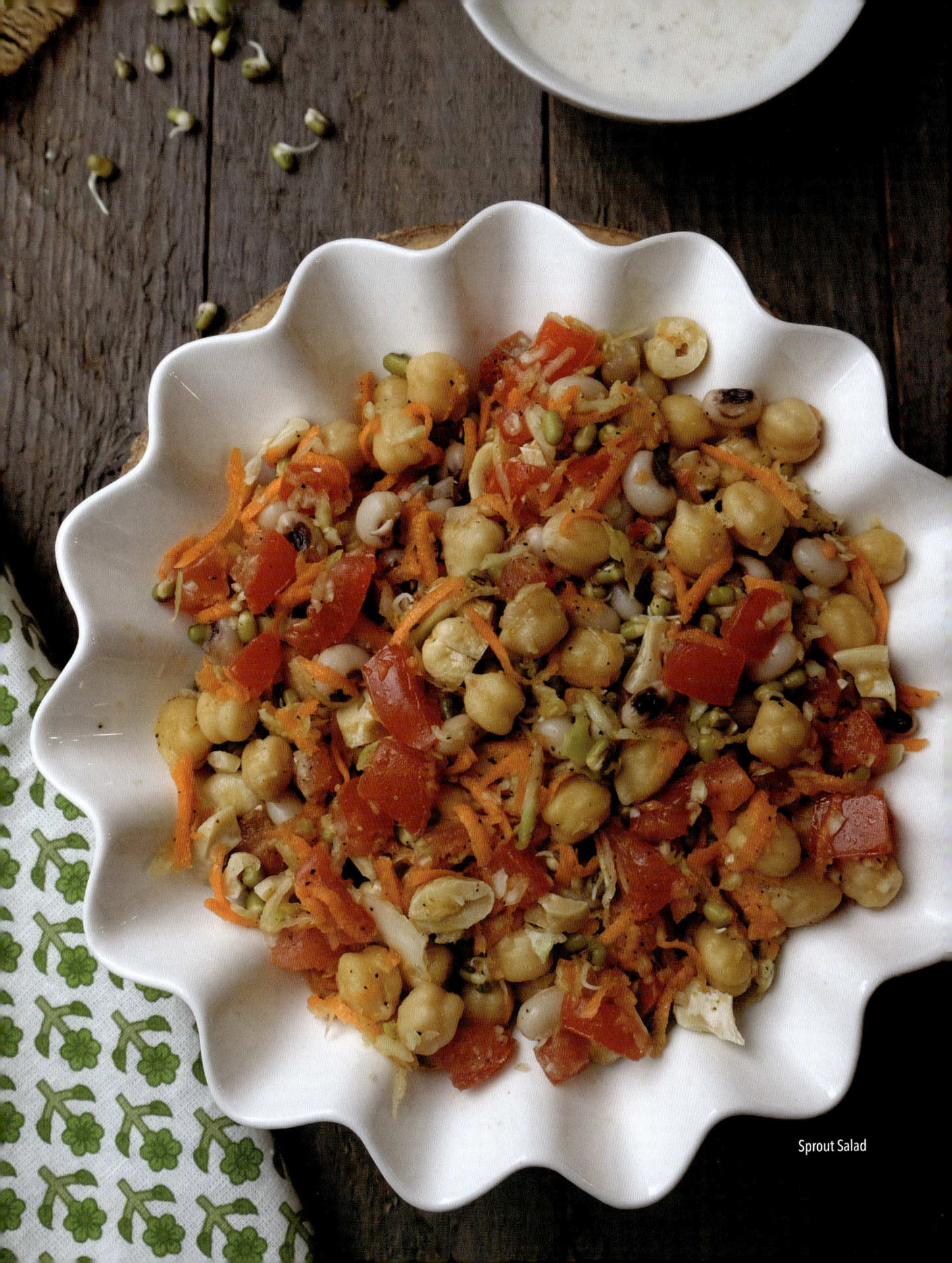

Sprout Salad

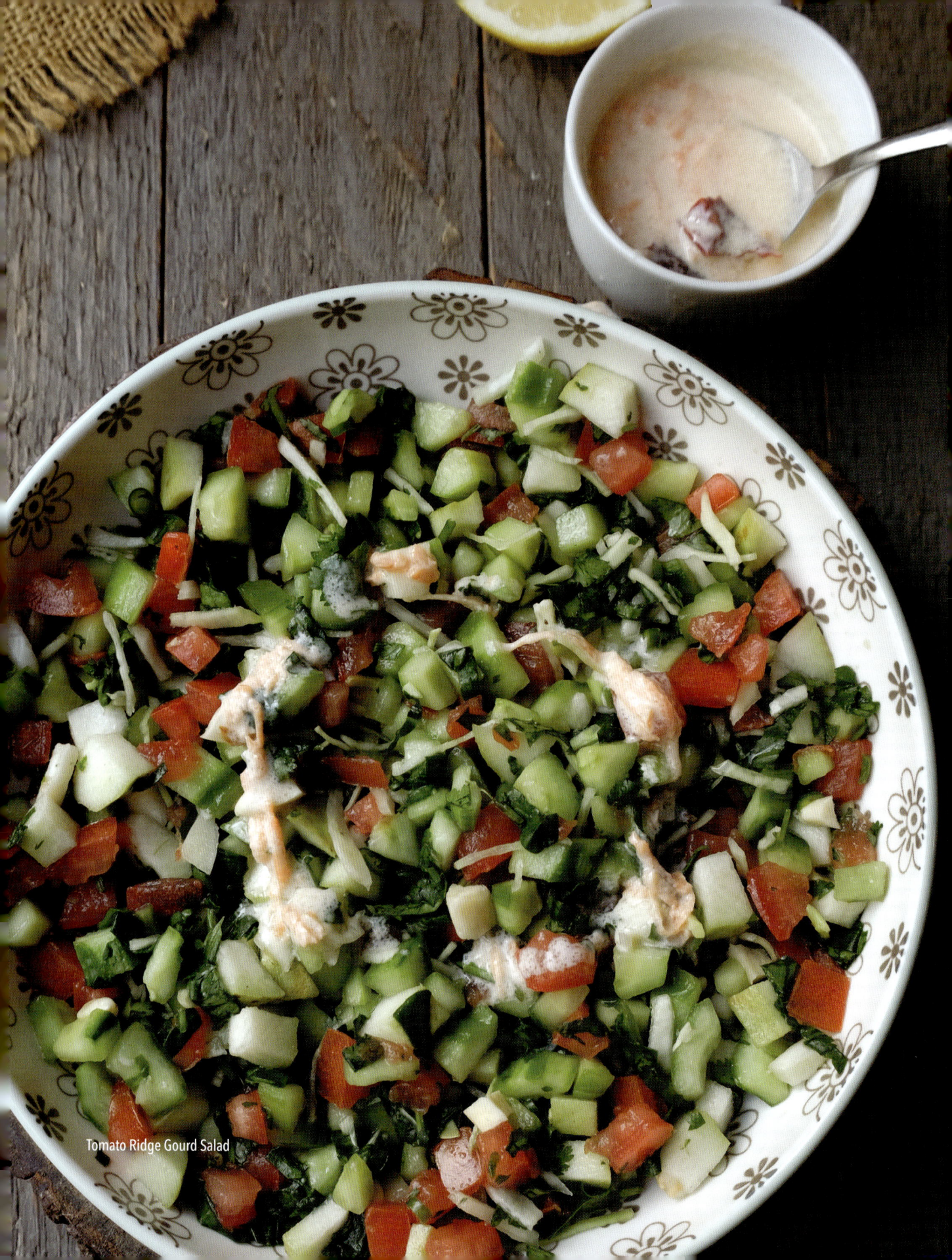

Tomato Ridge Gourd Salad

TOMATO RIDGE GOURD SALAD

Ingredients

Tomatoes (semi ripe): 6 oz. (160 ml),
cut into pieces

Ridge gourd (young): 6 oz. (160 ml),
cut into pieces

Cucumber: 6 oz. (160 ml)
cut into pieces

Spinach: 1.5 oz. (40 ml),
cut into pieces

Cabbage: 1.5 oz. (40 ml), grated

Coriander leaves: 1.5 oz. (40 ml),
cut into pieces

Soaked almonds: 1 teaspoon, thinly chopped

Available fruits (guava/green mango): 3 oz.
(80 ml)

Green chilis: 1.5 oz. (40 ml), cut into pieces

Salt: sufficient

Oil: 2 teaspoons

Directions

Put all the ingredients into a bowl and mix thoroughly. Top it with any of the seven dressings and eat the salad, slowly chewing it and enjoying its taste. I suggest the carrot dressing for this salad.

MIXED SALAD

Ingredients

Sprouted green gram: 3 oz. (80 ml)

Roasted white sesame: 1 teaspoon

Peas soaked for 12 hours: 1.5 oz. (40 ml)

Banana slices: 6 oz. (160 ml)

Guavas: 3 oz. (80 ml), chopped

Green tomatoes: 3 oz. (80 ml), chopped

Grated capsicum: 1.5 oz. (40 ml)

Coriander leaves: 1.5 oz. (40 ml), chopped

Lemon juice: 1 tablespoon

Dates: 3

Green chilis: 1.5 oz. (40 ml), chopped

Soaked almonds: 10

Oil: 4 teaspoons

Salt: sufficient quantity

Directions

Put all the ingredients into a bowl and mix thoroughly. Top it with any of the seven dressings and eat the salad, slowly chewing it and enjoying its taste. I suggest the chickpea dressing.

CABBAGE COCONUT SALAD

Ingredients

Cabbage: 3 oz. (80 ml) grated

Cucumber: 3 oz. (80 ml) grated

Unripe papaya: 3 oz. (80 ml) grated

Red capsicum: 3 oz. (80 ml) grated

Green chilis: 2

Soaked almonds: 10

Soaked peanuts: 10

Soaked sesame: 4 teaspoons

Lemon juice: 2 teaspoons

Salt: sufficient quantity

Honey: 1 tablespoon

Dates: 2

Oil: 2 tablespoons

Directions

Put all the ingredients into a bowl and mix thoroughly. Enjoy it with any of the seven dressings; however, I suggest the tamarind leaf dressing which suits this salad very well with its sour and sweet taste.

DRESSINGS

ALMOND DRESSING

Ingredients

Almonds: 20

Milk: 1.5 oz. (40 ml)

Salt: sufficient quantity

Sunflower oil: 2 tablespoons

Lemon juice: 2 tablespoons

Dry red chili flakes: 1½ tablespoons

White sesame powder: 2 teaspoons

Mustard seed powder: ½ teaspoon

Directions

Soak the almonds for 12 hours, peel them, and then grind them by adding milk and salt, in a mixie. Then add sunflower oil, lemon juice, dry red chili flakes, sesame powder, and mustard powder. This almond dressing can make any salad mouth-watering.

CHICKPEA DRESSING

Ingredients

Chickpeas: 3 oz. (80 ml)

Flax seeds: 1 tablespoon

White sesame: 1 tablespoon

Milk: 6 oz. (160 ml)

Sunflower oil: 2 tablespoons

Lemon juice: 2 tablespoons

Salt: sufficient quantity

Green chilis: 4, cut into pieces

Directions

Soak chickpeas for 12 hours, then boil them and grind them. Next, grind sesame seeds and flax seeds, adding milk and sunflower oil into a smooth paste. Next, mix it with the chickpea paste. Add lemon juice, salt, and green chilis cut into pieces.

This hot and sour dressing is ready to make your salad simply yummy.

COCONUT MILK DRESSING

Ingredients

Coconut: 1

Cashew nuts: 5

Mustard seeds: ½ teaspoon

Sunflower oil: 2 tablespoons

Lemon juice: 2 tablespoons

White sesame: 1 tablespoon

Green chilis: 2, cut into pieces

Salt: sufficient quantity

Directions

Break the coconut open and remove the meat. Or buy fresh coconut pieces, equal to the quantity of one coconut. Grind the coconut meat with a good amount of water and filter the paste. This produces coconut milk.

Next, grind the cashew nuts and mustard seeds, adding the coconut milk and oil. Finally, add lemon juice, white sesame, green chilis cut into pieces and salt.

Adding this dressing to a salad makes it mouth-watering.

YOUNG TAMARIND LEAF DRESSING

Ingredients

Young tamarind leaves: 12 oz. (320 ml)

Cashew nuts: 20

Ginger: small piece

Black peppers: 12

Green chilis: 2

Salt: sufficient quantity

Sunflower Oil: 1 tablespoon

Directions

Wash young tamarind leaves in water. Then grind them along with cashew nuts, ginger, black pepper, green chilis, and salt. Add the oil to the mixture to produce this dressing.

GREEN TOMATO DRESSING

Ingredients

Green tomatoes: 3, chopped

Groundnuts: 1.5 oz. (40 ml)

Almonds: 1.5 oz. (40 ml)

Dry red chilis: 3, cut into pieces

Green chilis: 2, cut into pieces

Sunflower Oil: 2 tablespoons

Onions: 6 oz. (160 ml), cut into pieces

Black pepper: 1 teaspoon

Coriander: 3 oz. (80 ml), chopped

Salt: sufficient quantity

Directions

Soak the groundnuts and almonds for 8 hours and set them aside.

Fry the dry red chilis in oil. Add the green tomatoes and roast them until the rawness goes.

Finally, grind all the ingredients including salt to produce a hot, sour and salty green tomato dressing to add taste to your salad.

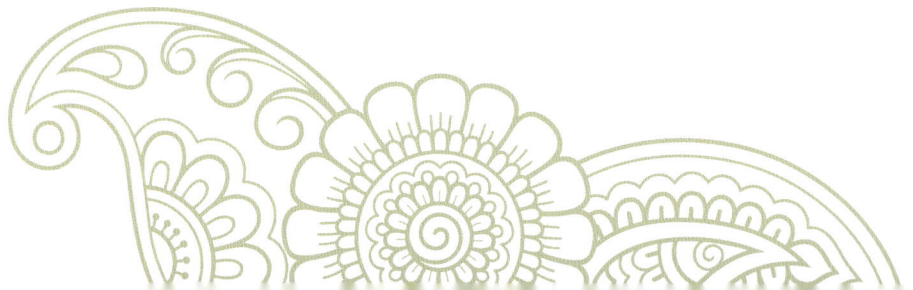

CARROT DRESSING

Ingredients

Coconut: 1

Grated carrot: 12 oz. (320 ml)

Coconut milk: 6 oz. (160 ml)

Dry red chilis: 4, cut into pieces

Lemon juice: 2 tablespoons

Salt: sufficient quantity

Sunflower oil: 1 tablespoon

Directions

Break a coconut into pieces, remove the meat and grind it, adding a good amount of water. Then, filter it to get coconut milk.

Mix the grated carrot and dry red chilis cut into pieces, adding in the coconut milk. Add lemon juice, oil and salt, and your marvelous carrot dressing gets ready.

YELLOW CUCUMBER DRESSING

Ingredients

Yellow cucumber: 1

Grated coconut: 3 oz. (80 ml)

Dry red chilis: 3

Curd (yogurt): 6 oz. (160 ml)

Salt: sufficient quantity

Sunflower Oil: 1 tablespoon

Directions

Fry the peeled and cut yellow cucumber in a tablespoon of oil until the rawness goes. Then grind it along with the grated coconut and the dry red chilis, adding the curd, salt, and oil to make it semi-thick. Use this dressing with any salad.

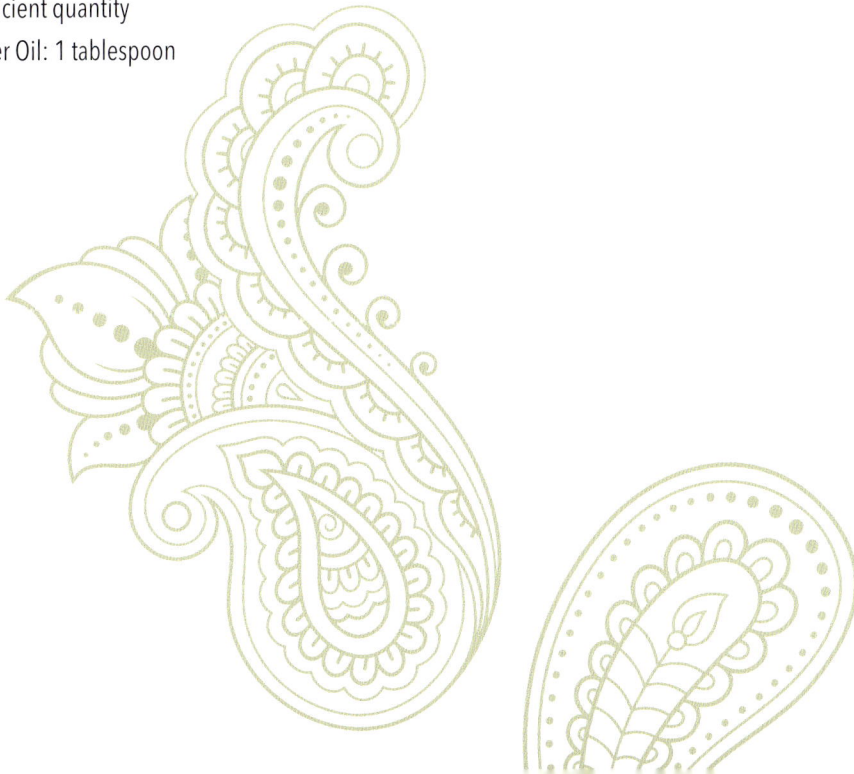

PART 2

12 EASY DO-AT-HOME EXERCISES

CONDITION YOUR BODY AND COUNTERACT HIGH BLOOD SUGAR

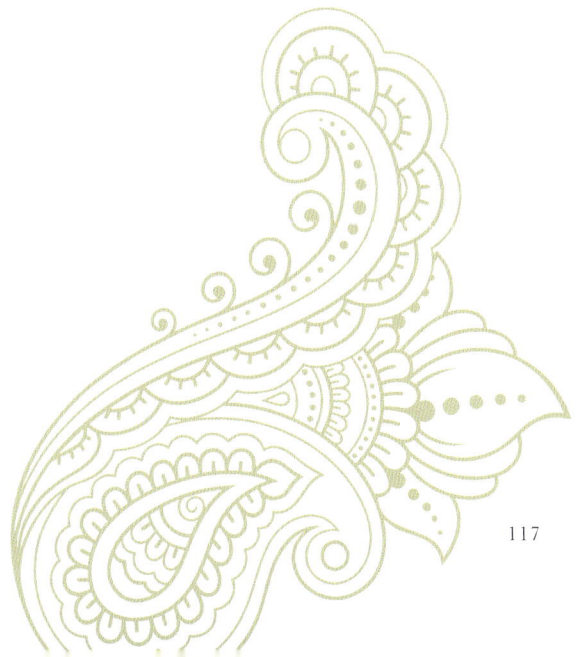

Exercising to Prevent Falls As You Age

Exercise offers tremendous benefits for everyone, but especially for people with diabetes or other chronic illnesses. Physical exercise helps condition your muscles and lubricate your joints, which improves your mobility. In addition, doing daily physical activity, even for just 30 minutes, helps you sleep and feel better, reduces anxiety, and improves your memory. Most importantly, exercise increases blood circulation to your brain.

If you have not been in the habit of exercising, you may find it hard to start a regular routine, especially a structured one. But there is a good reason to consider starting consistent, regular exercise activity: preventing falls. Statistics show that falls are the main cause of injury, disability, and death in the elderly. It has been estimated that more than one-third of persons 65 years or older fall each year, due to any number of causes, from simple tripping on the sidewalk to slipping in the bathtub or shower. But you can also experience falls due to the improper working of the balancing mechanism located in the inner ear, or impairment of your vision or depth perception, due to some type of limitation of your brain's signal processing mechanism or due to medication side effects.

The best way to decrease the chance of falling is to maintain as normal a balance and gait as possible. This requires good muscle tone, comfortable joint motion, and awareness of your surroundings. To achieve those, you need proper nerve function along with adequate concentration; these are necessary to make movement adjustments based on continuous input from your inner ears (where one's sense of equilibrium comes from) regarding your body in motion. You also need good vision that provides awareness of your surroundings.

The exercises I am suggesting are designed to be practiced in place and do not involve walking around. Rather than increasing the possibility of a fall, as you may be concerned about, these exercises will go a long way to preventing one.

The Many Other Benefits of Exercise

Before you peruse or begin trying the exercises, take some time now to read the following sections on the many benefits of regular exercise. These include improving your general well-being, muscle stability, joint mobility, and even your brain function. In addition, I will discuss the benefits regarding heart health and lung conditioning. Furthermore, according to the CDC, among adults aged 45 to 64 in the United States, 44% have pre-diabetes or diabetes, so I also point out how exercise can help lower blood sugar, though you cannot expect exercise alone to prevent the progression of pre-diabetes to Type 2 diabetes! That requires altering your diet, which is the goal of the recipes in this book.

General well-being

It is known that physical activity can help you sleep better and feel better. It can reduce the risk of twenty chronic health conditions, including heart disease and some cancers.

Exercise, in this context, is defined as any activity done to maintain and improve physical health and mental well-being. You can exercise outdoors or indoors. Outdoor exercises include walking, running, cycling, swimming, rowing, hiking, or playing sports; indoor exercises include dancing, weight or interval training, or skipping rope. There are many choices! Clearly, some of these can be done either outside or inside, either alone or in the company of others. Dynamic exercises such as running can improve your blood circulation, whereas static exercises such as weightlifting can increase your muscle strength as well as your blood pressure.

While the type of exercise can be tailored based on your goal and age, doing any exercise is better than doing none. In fact, the psychological and physiological benefits of adhering to an exercise routine are more pronounced when you recognize the value of exercise and voluntarily embrace it.[1] Daily exercise lasting at least 30 minutes has been shown to reduce anxiety and improve memory.

It has been clearly demonstrated that persons who remain sedentary have a higher risk of cardiovascular disease, such as heart attack and stroke, compared to those who exercise and expend at least 700 kcal (calories) of energy per week. According to the US Centers for Disease Control and Prevention, people who are physically active for about 150 minutes a week have a 33% lower risk of dying from all causes than those who are physically inactive.[2] This means that by exercising about 30 minutes each day of the week, you can significantly cut your risk of dying prematurely.

A recent study showed that for every 2,000 steps you take each day, your risk for premature death may fall by 8 to 11 percent.[3]

Muscle stability

As we get older, metabolic activities inside each cell in the body produce agents known as "Reactive Oxygen Species" (ROS) that can cause damage to proteins and/or genes.

1. Kennedy AB, Resnick PB (May 2015). "Mindfulness and Physical Activity". *American Journal of Lifestyle Medicine*. 9 (3): 3221–3323. doi:10.1177/1559827614564546. S2CID 73116017.

2. cdc.gov/physicalactivity/basics/pa-health/index.htm

3. Prospective Associations of Daily Step Counts and Intensity With Cancer and Cardiovascular Disease Incidence and Mortality and All-Cause Mortality. Borja del Pozo Cruz, PhD1; Matthew N. Ahmadi, PhD2; I-Min Lee, MBBS, ScD3,4; et al. *JAMA Intern Med.* Published online September 12, 2022. doi:10.1001/jamainternmed.2022.4000

For example, the atrophy of skeletal muscles that causes them to perform less efficiently is thought to be due to increased production of ROS. Regular muscle activity keeps the metabolic pathways working efficiently while reducing the production of ROS.

The importance of muscle function becomes clear when you consider a potentially life-threatening situation that necessitates your immediate movement, such as jumping out of the way of a car or walking through a crowd. With conditioned muscles that work with more efficiency than unconditioned ones, you can react and move faster.

To clearly understand the concept of muscle conditioning, it helps to know something about muscles in general and how they function in particular. A skeletal muscle contains multiple bundles composed of three different types of fibers, each based on distinct metabolic, contractile, and motor unit properties. The primary function of muscle is contraction. When a muscle contracts, the fibers release signaling molecules believed to be responsible for the health benefits of exercise. Another major contribution from muscle function is maintaining your body's stable internal temperature. During metabolic activities needed to produce ATP—the fuel that cells need to perform their internal operations—a lot of potential energy is lost as heat. In this process, every cell contributes to body heat, but the metabolic activity of muscles is responsible for 85% of it. You can see the critical part muscles play in providing heat when you shiver in extreme cold, as your muscles are attempting to generate heat.

Aerobic exercises of long duration such as running, swimming, and dancing require a steady supply of oxygen to generate ATP within cells. Anaerobic exercises such as sprinting and weightlifting are usually of shorter duration, during which ATP is produced through the breakdown of glucose without using much oxygen. Although glucose gives you a sudden spurt of energy, it can also result in the formation of lactic acid, which, when accumulated inside muscle fibers, can inhibit the ATP formation that you need for longer duration exercise. However, muscle conditioning can mitigate this by building more blood vessels to drain the acid. Most common exercises are partially aerobic and anaerobic.

Muscle strength comes from your muscle size, the strength of the nerve signals reaching the muscle, and mechanical factors such as joint capabilities, as well as the training you do to build muscle size. Although the number of muscle fibers cannot be increased through exercise, muscle can grow larger by adding new protein filaments alongside existing muscle cells. However, this may prove to be difficult to maintain as one gets older. In fact, muscle strength and the stamina for sustained physical activities both decline with age, largely due to the reduction in hormone levels and accumulation of damages to genes.

Joint mobility

The human skeleton, composed of 270 bones at birth, is the internal scaffolding that makes it possible for a person to stand, sit, and move around on two feet. The bones are composed mostly of calcium minerals and reach their maximum density around age 21. Your bones are about 14% of your total body weight.

Where two bones meet, a joint is created that connects the bones into a functional unit that allows for different types and degrees of movement. Some joints—such as knee, elbow, and shoulder—are self-lubricating. But injury, infection, surgery, or prolonged nonuse can result in a condition called fibrosis that limits the joint lubrication and thus the joint's function. Now you can understand the importance of regular exercise in maintaining joint functionality and the physical capability of the body.

Brain function

Each behavior you have consists of an input that triggers it, then nerve impulses that go through the brain to process it, and finally an output that manifests itself in your actions. Doing physical exercise follows the same general principle of input, processing, and output. Exercise thus helps keep your brain functioning, which can add to your alertness as you age.

One evidence of the importance of exercise for the brain is the finding that declining mental functions are almost twice as common among adults who are inactive as those who are active.[4]

In addition, people with high blood sugar had more than twice the risk of developing dementia than those without it. Persistent elevation of blood glucose could lead to glucose attaching to proteins and thus creating "advanced glycation end products" that are thought to be responsible for interfering with brain functions.[5] This means that if you are diabetic, physical activity is one of the best means of preventing deterioration of your brain function.

Ideally, most adults should get at least 150 minutes of moderate intensity physical activity on a weekly basis. This does not mean that the activity has to be uninterrupted. It can be broken into smaller segments such as 30 minutes a day. Even a simple exercise such as walking between 3,800 and 9,800 steps each day can reduce your risk of mental decline.[6]

---

4. Cross-sectional association between physical activity level and subjective cognitive decline among US adults aged ≥45 years. 2015 Preventive Medicine,Volume 141, December 2020, 106279 John D. Omura, David R. Brown, Lisa C. McGuire, et al.

5. Aragno, M.; Mastrocola, R. Dietary sugars and endogenous formation of advanced glycation end products: Emerging mechanisms of disease. *Nutrients* 2017, *9*, 385.

6. Association of Daily Step Count and Intensity With Incident Dementia in 78,430 Adults Living in the UK. Borja del Pozo Cruz, PhD1; Matthew Ahmadi, PhD2; Sharon L. Naismith, PhD3; et al. *JAMA Neurol.* Published online September 6, 2022. doi:10.1001/jamaneurol.2022.2672

Blood sugar control

Muscles can use either glucose or fatty acids as their fuel to produce the energy needed for exercising. Based on the type of meal you eat and how digestible the food components are that you consume, your blood sugar levels will start spiking about 60 to 90 minutes after eating. This corresponds with the release of insulin from the pancreas, which informs cells of the presence of glucose outside the cell wall.

The gene in charge of glucose acquisition then activates "transporters" that move to the cell wall to pick up the glucose molecules outside and bring them in. However, the quantity of insulin released matches the level of the spike in blood glucose only up to a point. This could be due to the presence of fatty acids in the bloodstream, which inform the pancreas about the availability of an alternative fuel, cutting the further release of insulin.

Your skeletal muscles burn roughly 90 mg of glucose each minute during continuous physical activity. This is to be expected because physical activity dominates the body's use of energy. Therefore, exercising immediately after a meal provides glucose from carbohydrates in the meal and insulin released from the pancreas that aids muscle glucose uptake. In addition, a muscle warmed by exercise has been found to activate transporters that can bring in more glucose even when insulin is not present outside. In short, people with diabetes can benefit by just taking a walk right after a meal. However, for exercise to be of practical use in controlling blood sugar, one has to be prepared to exercise after every carbohydrate-containing meal, as well as able to adjust the duration of exercise corresponding to the carbohydrate intake. I submit that both of these are not practical in daily life.

Even just standing up for a few minutes throughout the day and after meals can lower blood glucose on average by 9.5%. However, the best option is to walk two to five minutes every 30 minutes throughout the day, which will result in better glucose control. Keep in mind, however, you might develop an increased appetite following exercise, which could offset your attempt at glucose control.[7]

The most effective exercise, however, is between meals, even though your blood insulin level is at its lowest. In these situations, cellular energy production is influenced by three other hormones: glucagon, epinephrine, and growth hormone. When you exercise, your muscles send a message to the brain requesting additional fuel. The brain, in turn, sends signals to cause the release of these additional hormones. Glucagon stimulates the release of stored glucose from the liver, while epinephrine and growth hormone stimulate the release of fatty

7. The Acute Effects of Interrupting Prolonged Sitting Time in Adults with Standing and Light-Intensity Walking on Biomarkers of Cardiometabolic Health in Adults: A Systematic Review and Meta-analysis. Aidan J. Buffey, Matthew P. Herring, Christina K. Langley, et al. *Sports Medicine* 52:1765–1787 (February 2022)

acids from fat cells. The release of glucose from the liver helps maintain your blood glucose level so that nerves in the brain can function, while muscles rely on the fatty acids for their energy production. The use of released fatty acids from fat cells is why exercise can help you lose weight, albeit very small amounts are lost during an exercise routine.

But note that this metabolic fact means that in the long term, the availability of fatty acids ultimately determines the level of blood sugar control you can achieve from exercise. As you get older, and you are unable to maintain the same level of physical activity, you tend to gain weight from fat cells while losing muscle fiber from reduced exercise.

Heart health

The heart is a four-chambered pump made of muscle. It is responsible for sending blood to all parts of the body. The left ventricle sends blood carrying nutrients and oxygen to every cell in the body. The aorta is the main vessel that carries blood from the left ventricle. Branches of the aorta—the arteries—supply blood to every part of the body. Arteries further subdivide into smaller blood vessels called capillaries. Along the capillary walls are perforations, or tiny holes, that allow the fluid part of blood carrying nutrients—but not the red blood cells—to leak into the outside and reach nearby cells. (However, red cells can get out when there is injury to the capillary wall, causing bleeding. White blood cells can also get out when openings are created in the capillary wall by enzymes released during inflammation.)

The fluid leaking out from the blood allows each cell to pick up needed nutrients, as cells absorb whichever nutrients they need based on their functional specialization. In turn, cells discharge waste and carbon dioxide into blood carried by veins to return to the right side of the heart. Veins empty the blood into the right ventricle, which pumps the blood to the lungs where carbon dioxide is released into the air and oxygen is picked up. The oxygenated blood returns to the left side of the heart to repeat the cycle.

Regular exercise provides two benefits for the heart. On the one hand, it improves the supply of oxygen and nutrients, which increases the efficiency of the heart muscle. On the other hand, it conditions your heart muscle, which can then pump more blood with less effort compared to an unconditioned heart. In other words, systematic use of the heart makes heart muscles more efficient in their pumping performance. This means that you can have a lower number of heart beats in the long run, which can prolong the life of your heart muscle.

Lung conditioning

Every human being has to overcome an unavoidable challenge to survive on the earth: adapting to living in an environment of air, not water as it did in the womb. Before birth, a baby is surrounded by water, protected from the elements, and getting nourishment and oxygen fed through the umbilical cord. It is lulled into a state of meditation by the rhythmic beat of the mother's heart. Then at some moment, it is suddenly thrust into the unfamiliar medium of air and forced to acquire oxygen and nutrients by itself.

Taking a breath is the first act the baby performs, and the difficulty of that is evidenced in the cry heard during inhalation and exhalation of its first breath of air through the mouth. The air moving through the bronchial tubes displaces the water that until now has been keeping the air sacs at the end of the breathing tubes filled. From that first breath onward, the air sacs are meant to be kept open so that carbon dioxide produced during metabolic activities in the body can be exchanged for oxygen from the outside air.

Considering the importance of oxygen to life, nature made breathing to be automatic, though there is also some fine tuning of it in the control centers located in the brain. Based on the need for oxygen during different metabolic activities, the brain can increase the number of breaths per minute, such as during physical exercise. Movement of air into the lungs is accomplished by the action of muscles that expand the chest cavity, while moving air out is independent of skeletal muscle contraction, as it is accomplished by the contraction of fibers lining the air sacs that were stretched by the air during inhalation.

It is well known that for breathing to be effective, air passages have to be open; so the structural integrity of air sacs must thus be maintained. Chronic inflammation of the air sacs—such as that from smoking, inhalation of asbestos particles, and infections from bacteria and fungi—can impede air flow and the oxygenation of blood, either by narrowing the air passages or by reducing the efficiency of the exchange of air in the air sacs.

Here is a simple exercise that can improve the conditioning of chest wall muscles and that of the fibers of the air sacs. Try this exercise to strengthen the muscles involved in air movement.

Simple Deep Breathing Exercise

1. Sit comfortably with your legs firmly planted.
2. Take a deep breath to a mental count of four.
3. Hold the breath for a mental count of five.
4. Purse your lips and force the air through the lips to a mental count of twenty or more.

Repeat this exercise as many times as you are comfortable and as often as time permits. See below for another exercise routine using deep breathing that can also help you condition the fibers lining the air sacs.

Instructions for the Easy Exercises

Here are 12 different exercises, and each has an accompanying animated video showing you how to do it. You can access the videos by clicking the QR code next to the exercise title. These exercises are easy to execute in the comfort of your home, at any time you feel the desire, to offset boredom or anxiety or simply put, when you have nothing else to do.

Note that you don't have to do all of them, or in the same sequence presented. However, I urge you to do one or more of these exercises whenever you get some free time. Some of them can be done anywhere and anytime. For example, when you are bored or when you are just sitting around on the couch, do the deep breathing exercise, paying attention to the movement of air through your nose and that of your chest wall muscles. Similarly, you can do the breathing exercise when you are listening to something on TV or during commercials, or when you are waiting for service in a restaurant or any other similar situation.

Toe taps are an excellent activity when you are a passenger in a car, train, or airplane, or when there is a dull moment while you are sitting, watching a stage event or sport, during a meeting or while waiting for an appointment. You could also do toe taps in the standing position when you are forced to stand in a train, subway, slow moving commuter vehicle, using one leg after another.

You can do the leg-related exercises every morning before you get out of your bed. In fact, every time you lie down, you have an opportunity to do one or more of the leg exercises. If you have a history of feeling dizzy when you stand up suddenly after being on your back for some time, this could be due to a condition called postural hypotension. Doing leg exercises before getting up to a sitting position or doing toe tapping in the sitting position before standing up, could speed delivery of blood to your brain and limit the degree of dizziness from postural hypotension.

Over time, you may find other opportunities to put into practice these exercises. You may even want to invent new exercises based on these that you enjoy doing to keep your muscles, joints, and lungs functionally efficient.

Note: You should first get your doctor's or physical therapist's advice as to what types of exercises you can comfortably do. For example, if you are already out of shape and not yet limber, you may not be able to perform some of these exercises, especially those involving bending your back. Make sure the sofa or bed you use is strong enough to support you.

1. Dynamic arms sweep. To perform this exercise, stand upright with your feet hip-width apart resting comfortably on the ground. Sweep both hands to the left in the horizontal plane, keeping your elbows straight. Have your left palm facing forward, and your right palm facing upward. Gradually move both arms to the right, then back to the left. Increase the number of repetitions as you get more comfortable with the exercise.

2. Dynamic front arms. To perform this exercise, stand upright with your feet resting hip-width apart comfortably on the ground. While taking a deep breath, spread your arms to their respective sides, with elbows straight and palms facing forward. While exhaling, gradually move both arms to meet the palms in front of you. Open the arms again to the sides. Repeat the exercise at least three times. Increase the number of repetitions as you get more comfortable with the exercise.

3. Dynamic top arms. To perform this exercise, stand upright with your feet resting hip-width apart comfortably on the ground. Spread your arms to their respective sides in the horizontal plane with elbows straight and palms facing upward. Gradually move both arms to meet palms above your head. Open the arms again and repeat the exercise at least three times. Increase the number of repetitions as you get more comfortable with the exercise.

4. Deep breathing exercise. To perform this exercise, sit on a sofa or the bedside, with your feet resting comfortably on the ground. Rest your hands on your thighs, palms facing upwards. Bend your fingers so that the thumb touches the tip of your index (pointer) finger. Holding that position, take a deep breath through your nose to a silent count of four. Hold your breath to a silent count of five. Exhale through your nose to a silent count of six. Then hold your breath and relax to a silent count of seven. Repeat the exercise three more times, with the thumb touching each of the other three fingers in sequence.

5. Shoulder stretch. To perform this exercise, sit upright on a sofa or bedside with your legs resting comfortably on the ground. Keep your hands with palms together in front of your legs. Bend your head gently as far down as you can with your fingers pointing down. Then, keeping one hand pointing down as far as you can go, lift and move the other hand up over your head as far back as possible to stretch your shoulder. Gently reverse the movement to bring your hand back down to the floor as much as possible. Repeat the exercise using the other hand, then repeat stretching with both hands together over the head. Repeat the whole routine at least three times. Increase the number of repetitions as you get more comfortable with the exercise,

6. Toe taps. To perform this exercise, sit on a sofa or bedside with your feet resting comfortably on the ground. You may use any comfortable footwear or be barefoot. Lift the right leg a few inches, point your toes down, and swing your foot backwards. Tap your toes as you move your foot forwards until you can go no further. Then tap back to the starting position and put your heel down. Then do the exercise with your left foot. Repeat the exercise three times and increase the number of repetitions as you get more comfortable with the exercise.

7. Deadbugs. To perform this exercise, lie flat on your back on the floor, or on a sofa or bed, with your palms facing down at your side. If necessary, you may use a pillow under your knees. Bend one knee upwards, then stretch the leg back down. Repeat the process using the other leg. Then, repeat the same activity with both knees bent at the same time, using your hands to gently pull your knees down towards your stomach. Repeat the exercise at least three times. Increase the number of repetitions as you get more comfortable with the exercise.

8. V-ups. To perform this exercise, lie flat on your back on the floor, or on a sofa or bed, with your palms facing down at your side. Lift your head up and extend your hands over your legs to get your fingertips towards your toes as far as you can go. You may bend your knee as you stretch your hands forward. Immediately lay your head back down while bringing your arms back. Repeat the exercise at least three times. Increase the number of repetitions as you get more comfortable with the exercise.

9. Leg lift. To perform this exercise, lie flat on your back on the floor, or on a sofa or bed, with your palms facing down.

Lift one leg from your hip in the fully extended position without bending the knee by a few inches and immediately put it down. Repeat the same with the other leg. Then lift both legs up together in the fully extended position by a few inches. Immediately bring the legs down together. Repeat the exercise at least three times. Increase the number of repetitions as you get more comfortable with the exercise.

10. Shoulder stand. You should be careful when doing this exercise; otherwise you could hurt your back. To perform this exercise, lie flat on your back on the floor, or on a sofa or bed, with your palms facing down. Lift both legs up together in the fully extended position, bending at your hip joint while keeping your knees straight. Lift your hips up and support your back with your palms to help keep your legs as vertical as possible. Your body will be almost in an L-shape. Hold that position to a mental count of ten. Increase the duration of holding your legs up as you get more comfortable with the exercise.

11. Air cycle. To perform this exercise, lie flat on your back on the floor, or on a sofa or bed, with your palms facing down at your side. Lift both legs up together in the fully extended position, bending at your hip joint while keeping your knees straight. Lift your hips up and support your back with your palms to help keep your legs as vertical as possible. Your body will be almost in an L-shape. While holding that position, move your feet and legs as if you were bicycling to a mental count of ten. Increase the duration of air cycling as you get more comfortable with the exercise.

12. Leg flip. To perform this exercise, lie flat on your back on the floor, or on a sofa or bed. Lift both legs up together in the fully extended position, bending at your hip joint while keeping your knees straight. Lift your hips up, supporting your back with your palms if needed. Keep moving your legs as far back as possible, bringing your toes over your head. Your body will be almost in a U-shape. Reverse the movement slowly until your heels are back on the sofa. Repeat the exercise at least three times. Increase the number of repetitions as you get more comfortable with the exercise.

EPILOGUE

It would be natural for you to allow your fear of yet another failure to hold you back from adopting new eating and exercise habits. But as long as your intention is clear and precise, it can help you follow your chosen path to your goal. Go over the plan in your mind periodically and visualize how you can overcome the difficulties in front of you. Do not allow yourself to be discouraged by one day of overeating or going off your promise to eat healthy foods.

The more you discover your inner strength, the more confident you will become. Remind yourself that before you were diagnosed with Type 2 diabetes, you lived, perhaps for many decades, having normal blood sugar levels. It was not a change in your genetic makeup that made you diabetic during your midlife but a change in your lifestyle. And that is something that is completely within your control.

To help you keep your motivation to establish a new lifestyle related to modifying your diet and exercise habits, let me suggest the following five steps. But keep in mind that your motivation becomes real only when it comes from within you. In this connection, let me tell you that I have two objectives in writing this book. The first is to help YOU learn how to reduce the total food energy you consume by concentrating on the enjoyment of eating. Nature gives us a clue by putting all the nutrients an adult body needs into natural packages: vegetables, fruits, nuts, and other edibles that require chewing. The more you chew, the greater percentage of each bite of food you will enjoy; additionally, your own control centers inform you when to stop eating that food by reducing the intensity of enjoyment.

My second objective is to help you control your blood sugar level by reducing your intake of glucose. For this you have to voluntarily replace grain-based foods with millets, quinoa, etc.

As for exercise, I am all for it; but not for control of blood sugar. I promote exercise as a way to condition the body for greater general health. Although exercise may work for some people in the early stages of Type 2 diabetes to burn glucose and lower their blood sugar, this degree of glucose reduction cannot be sustained by exercise, due to ageing-related loss of muscle strength. As you get older, you simply do not burn as much glucose when exercising.

Therefore, in addition to exercise and, or walking, I advise you, once again, to switch from your grain based-meals, which are full of carbohydrates to non-grain foods, i.e., foods with millets, quinoa, brown rice, etc. as shown in the recipe part of the book, which have less carbohydrate content, with the result that you will begin freeing yourself from not only diabetes by controlling your blood sugar levels but also from medications resulting in unnecessary complications as well as the loss of money. Simultaneously you will control your weight also.

INDEX OF RECIPES

ACKNOWLEDGMENTS

Dr. John Poothullil

I thank D.C. Hanumantharao, whose delicious recipes are the backbone of this book. I thank my publishers, Rick Benzel and Susan Shankin, for making such a book happen and for their excellent work in editing and designing it. Thanks also to the following people who have contributed to the book in many ways:

- Maya Mohan for the preparation, display, and photographs of foods.
- Darcy Hughes and Felipe Zamora for their promotional marketing work.
- Elizabeth Lenthall for her assistance in helping with this cookbook including the cover design.
- Dr. K. R. Raju, Dr. Kantilal, Dr. Ch. S. R. B. Deekshithulu, Mr. A. Rambabu, and Sophia LaValle for their testimonials
- My wife of 50 years, Maria Poothullil, for her patience and support as I endeavor to challenge the theory of insulin resistance and propose a new way to explain the real cause of Type 2 diabetes and the right cure through my books and speaking engagements.

D. C. Hanumantharao

First, I express my heartfelt gratitude to my wife, Padmavathi, and my daughter-in-law, Priyanka Sandhya, for encouraging me to write a book with diabetes-friendly recipes so that those suffering from the complication may benefit from it.

I convey my deep sense of thankfulness to my friends in Portland, Mr. Ravji Patel, Mrs. Reena, and Mr. Ajith for their support and technical guidance in the preparation of the book.

I will be failing in my duty if I miss acknowledging my indebtedness to Dr. John M. Poothullil, a renowned physician, for asking me to suggest recipes beneficial to people with diabetes, and his regular inputs and suggestions during the making of the book. I always remember him with respect for his noble idea of bringing light into the lives of people suffering from diabetes by promoting non-grain foods to replace grain-based meals.

ABOUT THE AUTHORS

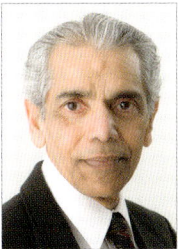

John M. Poothullil, MD, FRCP

Dr. Poothullil practiced medicine as a pediatrician and allergist for more than 30 years, with 27 of those years in the state of Texas. He received his medical degree from the University of Kerala, India in 1968, after which he completed two years of medical residency in Washington, D.C., and Phoenix, Arizona and two years of fellowship, one in Milwaukee, Wisconsin and the other in Ontario, Canada. He began his practice in 1974 and retired in 2008. He holds certifications from the American Board of Pediatrics, The American Board of Allergy & Immunology, and the Canadian Board of Pediatrics.

During his medical practice, John became interested in understanding the causes of and interconnections between hunger, satiation, and weight gain. His interest turned into a passion and a multi-decade personal study and research project that led him to read many medical journal articles, medical textbooks, and other scholarly works in biology, biochemistry, physiology, endocrinology, and cellular metabolic functions. This eventually guided Dr. Poothullil to investigate the theory of insulin resistance as it relates to diabetes. Recognizing that this theory was illogical, he spent several years rethinking the biology behind high blood sugar and developed the fatty acid burn theory as the real cause of diabetes.

He then continued researching the linkage between diabetes and cancer and developed additional insights into the causes of childhood and adult cancer and possible treatments involving low-carbohydrate diets to initiate starving of cancer cells by removing their main source of energy — glucose from grains.

Dr. Poothullil has written articles on hunger and satiation, weight loss, diabetes, and the senses of taste and smell. His articles have been published in medical journals such as *Physiology and Behavior, Neuroscience and Biobehavioral Reviews, Journal of Women's Health, Journal of Applied Research, Nutrition,* and *Nutritional Neuroscience.* His articles on diabetes have been published in *Alternative Medicine, Whole Person, India Abroad,* and several other magazines.

Dr. Poothullil is an active speaker on diabetes and cancer. He has appeared on four television shows, interviewed on over 60 national and local radio programs, and given more than 40 talks to groups in bookstores and private groups and associations. An interview with him appeared in the *Washington Post*. He has published nearly 130 blogs on his website DrJohnOnHealth.com.

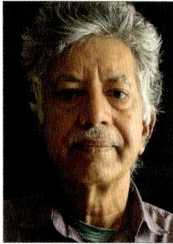

D. C. Hanumantharao

D. C. Hanumantharao, MA in English, Telugu, Sanskrit and Education & MPhil in English.

Sri D. C. Hanumantharao worked as an English lecturer and Principal of Sri Vasavi Kanyaka Parameswari & Pithani Venkanna Junior College, Penugonda, West Godavari District, Andhra Pradesh, for 35 years. After his retirement in 2012 he worked as Assistant professor of English in two Engineering Colleges in Hyderabad for another 8 years and quit his teaching career to live a hassle-free life. He has translated books and stories from Telugu to English and vice versa. He has given around 50 lectures in different workshops and seminars on English grammar, language and literature in various colleges in Andhra Pradesh and Telangana. He was awarded the State Best Teacher award in 2011.

He went to the USA along with his wife in 2021 to spend the rest of his life with his children. Now he is in Portland, where he has got acquainted with Dr. John M. Poothullil on whose request he translated the latter's book *Diabetes: The Real Cause and the Right Cure* from English to Telugu. The book has been published this year. He has also translated as many as ten articles of Dr. Poothullil on various medical topics from English to Telugu. He has also participated in TV interviews along with the same doctor on various channels in the two Telugu states. Now he has written this book in association with Dr. Poothullil and translated it into Telugu.

Sri Hanumantharao's deep study of books on Ayurveda and Naturopathy from the point of view of dietary therapy, i.e., modifying or adopting a diet to treat or prevent a disease, promote health or detoxify the body as well as his interaction with knowledgeable people in the field coupled with his own interest in helping patients, especially those suffering from Type 2 diabetes prompted him to bring out more than a hundred recipes for diabetes friendly meals, snacks and salads, which he has incorporated in the present book.

Currently, he is translating articles on different medical conditions written by Dr. Poothullil from English to Telugu, besides giving lectures on educational and spiritual matters.

OTHER BOOKS BY DR. POOTHULLIL

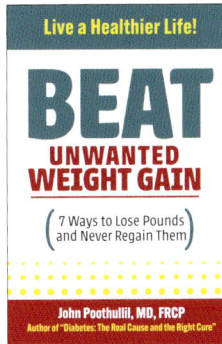

Beat Unwanted Weight Gain: 7 Ways to Lose Pounds and Never Regain Them

The last weight loss book you'll ever need! Struggling to lose weight and keep it off? Trying to recapture the body of your youth? This groundbreaking book is your ultimate guide to sustainable weight loss and reclaiming your energy and health.Dr. John M. Poothullil draws on decades of research to reveal the seven most essential strategies for shedding pounds and keeping them off for good.

Inside, you'll discover how to:

- Recognize and return to your "authentic" weight (the real you).
- Understand and overcome the triggers that lead you to overeat.
- Tune in to your body's real hunger and fullness signals.
- Break free from your unhealthy eating and food-shopping habits.
- Cut back on grain-based carbs, the real culprits in weight gain.
- Eat for better health, and to feel great.
- Embrace exercise as a tool for overall wellness—not just weight loss.

Packed with many "Aha" insights and actionable advice, this book will truly change the way you think about food, nutrition, and your body. Say goodbye to quick-fix solutions and dieting gimmicks. Instead, learn to nourish your body, achieve your healthiest weight, and rediscover the joy of living well.

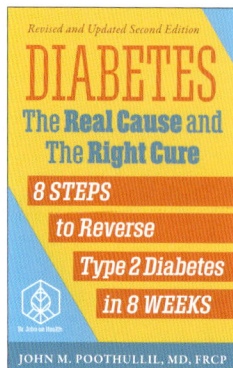

**Revised and Updated Second Edition
Diabetes—The Real Cause and The Right Cure:
8 Steps to Reverse Type 2 Diabetes in 8 Weeks**

If you have Type 2 diabetes, this book is a game-changer. Type 2 diabetes is fast becoming a global pandemic, affecting more than half a billion people worldwide—and that number is projected to double in the next 30 years. Most diabetics are treated with medications or insulin injections to "control" their diabetes, yet they still develop the complications of the condition. Diabetes is a major cause of kidney failure, loss of eyesight, heart attack, stroke, and amputation of lower limbs.

After 25 years of studying the cause and treatment of Type 2 diabetes, Dr. John Poothullil, MD, proposes that medical science has made a serious error—the theory of insulin resistance is incorrect. This has major implications.

From his research, Poothullil can show that diabetes is caused by the modern diet full of grains—including wheat, barley, rice, oats, corn, and the many products made with the flour of these grains. When people excessively consume grains, it fills their fat cells and eventually forces a normal body metabolism to go haywire, leaving glucose in the bloodstream. This causes high blood sugar, leading to Type 2 diabetes.

Finalist, 2017 Beverly Hills Book Awards, Diet & Nutrition Category.

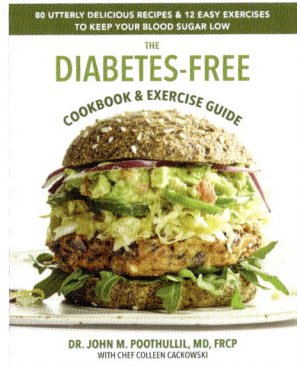

The Diabetes-Free Cookbook & Exercise Guide:
80 Utterly Delicious Recipes & 12 Easy Exercises to Keep Your Blood Sugar Low

Don't let Type 2 diabetes or pre-diabetes control your life—start a delicious new journey to a healthier, happier you today! Discover how you can live a diabetes-free life with Dr. John's groundbreaking cookbook and exercise guide. With over 80 appetizing low-carb recipes created by Chef Colleen Cackowski, you'll never miss the high-carb, high-sugar foods of your past. Every recipe nourishes your body and keeps your blood sugar levels in check so you can enjoy tasty, satisfying meals. Dr. John also offers 12 easy-to-do exercises to boost your flexibility and balance and keep you healthy as you age.

I know that reducing carbohydrates in the diet helps in better control of blood sugar. I can easily conclude that the methods advocated in this book by Dr. John will help in controlling Type 2 diabetes.
—Kuriakose Thekkethala M.D., FAAFP

Filled with tons of easy-to-make meals and encourages enjoyable meal planning for moms like me. I highly recommend this book to diabetics and families trying to live and eat healthily.
—Maria Chalissery, M.Sc., Diet Technician

If you are looking for ways to improve your health and add more zing to your meals, these recipes are exactly what you need.
—Jyoti Veeramoney, Chef, Certified Yoga Instructor

These exercises are great because they focus on dynamic movement that improves joint range of motion and flexibility. They require no equipment, build core strength and stabilization, and incorporate movements that can correct posture, which can decrease the risk of falling.
—Sophia LaValle, NASM Certified Personal Trainer

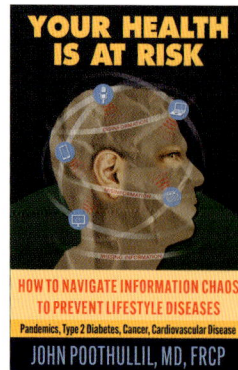

Your Health Is at Risk:
How to Navigate Information Chaos to Prevent Lifestyle.

Accurate health information can keep you free of lifestyle diseases! In this book, Dr. John Poothullil explains in detail how disinformation, misinformation, or missing information could lead you to lifestyle conditions, and suggests ways to use critical thinking to deal with them.

And when it comes to your health, DMMI can be especially dangerous. Don't fall victim to DMMI in your attempt to protect your health. Read this book and get sound, insightful advice and accurate, medical science-based information so you can make wise decisions about your lifestyle and healthcare.

This book is the best of its kind to guide you correctly and help you avoid mistakes that can harm you and your loved ones.   —Dr. Venugopal Menon, MD,
FAAP, FAAA&I, FACAA&I, Fellow of the Royal Society of Medicine, London

As a broadcaster, I've covered the consequences of disinformation and misinformation, especially regarding the COVID-19 pandemic. Dr. John's timely examination of DMMI is crucial to making informed, accurate decisions about your health.
                    —Matt Ray, Host of America's First News Radio Program

Gold Medal Winner, 2023 Nautilus Book Awards and Independent Press (Ippy) Awards.